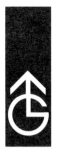

BABIES
& YOUNG
CHILDREN

Dr Chris Steele

*gives practical advice
and helpful information
on*

BABIES
& YOUNG
CHILDREN

Lennard Publishing
in association with
Granada Television and Prospect Pictures

Lennard Publishing
a division of
Lennard Associates Ltd
Mackerye End Harpenden
Herts AL5 5DR

British Library CIP Data is available

ISBN 1 85291 104 2

First published in 1991

This book accompanies the series
Babies and Young Children
made by Prospect Pictures for Granada Television
and transmitted for the first time
on the ITV network in October 1991

Design by Forest Publication Services, Luton.
Index program by Mark Stephenson
Cover design by Cooper Wilson
Cover origination by Amega Litho Ltd, London
Diagrams by Paul Cooper and Rob Shone

Photograph of the house dust mite on page 97
reproduced by kind permission of
Searle Consumer Products/Dr Matthew Colloff

Printed and bound in Great Britain
by Butler & Tanner Ltd, Fome and London

CONTENTS

INTRODUCTION

For all you Mums and Dads who want a simple, down to earth, commonsense approach to the medical problems of your 'little ones', here is an easy-to-read guide! You should be able to dip in and dip out of this book at will. It is not a lengthy tome, and you won't find it heavy going. In fact I hope you will pick up some interesting facts that you never knew before!

For the past three years between 1,000 and 2,000 people have called me every Thursday on a live medical phone-in on ITV's *This Morning* television programme. They have called to ask me for advice regarding their own medical problems or medical treatment. I hope that I have helped some of those callers, because over the years they have taught me one sad fact – that we doctors could be doing a far better job in listening to what our patients tell us and in explaining to our patients what is wrong with them. As a GP in a very busy practice I am probably as guilty as any of my colleagues in this respect. We all seem to have to cope with an ever-increasing workload in an ever-decreasing amount of time!

As doctors we should not only be treating our patients but we should be teaching them – teaching them not only about what their illness is, but also how best to manage that illness and, if possible, how best to prevent illness in general. This book endeavours to teach the reader about some of the more common problems that affect babies and young children. When your baby or child is unwell you want reassurance, and you need information about your child's illness.

This book explains, in language which I hope can be easily understood, the common disorders that affect babies and young children. It is not meant to be a comprehensive reference book covering every single disorder that your baby could possibly develop. As you will see, I have concentrated on many of the 'common or garden' problems such as nappy rash, crying babies, feeding difficulties etc. and also some of the more serious and distressing disorders such as asthma, eczema and the infectious diseases. I have tried to present the latest medical information on such problems as cot death, immunisation, allergic conditions and passive smoking.

To all Mums and to all females, I apologise! You will see as you read further that I have taken the outright liberty of referring to babies in this book as if they were all little boys! This has been done to make life easier for me, the writer, and also to make the text flow in an easier fashion. It looks messy and is awkward to read when you put 'he/she' throughout the text- and I do object to any baby or child being referred to as 'it'! So, ladies, do forgive me!

I make no apologies for any repetition that has occurred in the book. Some medical points are of such importance that they are well worth repeating, and some items of advice need to be reiterated time and time again. On a specific point I strongly recommend that, as soon as you have finished reading this introduction, you IMMEDIATELY read the section on choking and memorize it. I am not being alarmist, but if at any time a child (or adult for that matter) experiences a choking fit, you will not have time to turn to a book on how to cope with the emergency. Choking is rare, but when it happens it is a matter of extreme urgency – seconds count. If you know and remember the simple techniques shown on pages 135 and 136 you could save a life.

I do hope you find this book useful and an interesting read. I would love to receive your comments or queries, and indeed any recommendations for topics to be covered in future publications.

I wish you and your little ones the best of health!

Dr Chris Steele, M.B., Ch.B.
'This Morning'
Granada Television
Albert Dock
Liverpool L3 4AA

BABY PROBLEMS

BECOMING A PARENT

Your first child tends to be a source of great worry and concern. You don't know what is normal or abnormal, and as you have had no previous experience of bringing up a child everything that happens to your new baby is a first-time experience for you. So you don't know what to expect and, human nature being what it is, you tend to think the worst about every little symptom that your baby develops.

It certainly is easier bringing up a second child, through experience you know how to handle the problems, you know what is important and what is not worth worrying about. My wife and I have four children, and I can tell you it certainly gets a lot easier, despite the increased workload, as you become more experienced in raising a family. Without that experience it is difficult to get things into perspective. So with your first baby you will worry, you will lose sleep, and you'll get frights from time to time. This is a time when you have to turn to others for help, and don't be afraid ortoo proud to ask.

PROBLEMS WITH BABY?

If you are ever in doubt about what to do with your baby:

Firstly:
* Follow your natural instinct.
* Do what YOU feel is right, do what comes naturally.
* Use your common sense.

Then:
* Go to an EXPERIENCED parent:
  – your own mother or father
  – brothers and sisters who have families of their own
  – your friends who also have little ones.
* Go to reputable books on baby and child care.

Finally:
* Get in contact with any of these health professionals:
  – your midwife
  – your health visitor
  – your local child clinic
  – your practice nurse
  – your GP

FEEDING

A pregnant mother getting close to her delivery date, is faced with all sorts of dilemmas regarding the care of the new baby, especially if this baby is her first! All activities with her newborn will be new experiences for her, and so well-meaning individuals proffer their advice on feeding, bathing, clothing, sleeping, nappy-folding, the best powders and creams, etc., etc.

Caring for the new baby would appear to be a mine field of potential disasters for the inexperienced mum – it's not!

How many parents are there in this country? *A lot!*
How many of them have made disastrous mistakes in looking after their children? *Very few!*

Remember you've got your own natural instincts and also common sense on your side. You do, sometimes, hear peculiar advice given out, even from those who appear to be leading academic specialists. There's rarely a day goes by when I don't ask myself:

"WHATEVER HAPPENED
TO
COMMON SENSE?"

Let's now look at the feeding of your baby. One of the most perplexing and controversial issues is the following:

Question:
What sort of milk should I give my baby?

Answer:
Up to 6 months:
the baby should, if possible, be fed on breast milk.

> BREAST IS BEST!
> - see page 12.

If breast feeding is not possible for you, then *any* of the infant formula milks will do. They are well balanced feeds and there's little to choose between them.

* From 6–12 months – continue breast feeding. Babies on bottles should continue on infant formula, or change up to a follow-on milk, such as *Junior Milk* or *Progress*.

* Between 1 and 2 years. Either cow's milk or the follow-on milks. At this age, along with a mixed diet, both are acceptable. Skimmed and semi-skimmed milks are totally unacceptable, as their

10

energy content is far too low for the under 2 year-old.

COW'S MILK AND INFANTS

An infant is defined as a baby up to the age of 12 months.

Cow's milk is produced by the mother cow to feed HER baby, not your baby human! It contains everything her baby calf needs in its early months of development. It is not intended to be put into the tiny sensitive body of a baby from another species of animal – the human baby.

It can be harmful to give cow's milk to an infant and the foreign proteins in cow's milk can produce all sorts of problems to the growing baby.

* Ordinary cow's milk should NOT be given to babies under 12 months of age.

* Cow's milk contains insufficient vitamins for a baby under 1 year.

* Cow's milk contains insufficient iron for a baby under 1 year.

* Cow's milk can cause mild internal bleeding in the stomach and intestines in one third of infants!

* Cow's milk has higher concentrations of saturated fats and sodium than infant formulas.

* Infants fed on ordinary cow's milk during their first year of life are more prone to developing eczema, asthma, hay fever and other allergies.

* In particular, premature babies whose families have a history of eczema, asthma or hay fever, should never receive cow's milk in their first 12 months, as they are very specifically prone to developing those allergic diseases after exposure to the protein in cow's milk. Nor should they receive eggs until they are at least 9–12 months old.

TEN REASONS FOR BREAST FEEDING

1. It's what nature intended for your baby.
2. It provides the perfect balance of nutrients and energy for healthy growth. Breast-fed babies are rarely overweight.
3. It provides the baby with human hormones and other

11

active substances which are not present in other milks.

4. It provides the baby with antibodies from the mother to give him protection against infections and disease.
5. Breast-fed babies are less prone to gastroenteritis and, if they do get it, they recover quickly.
6. The concentration of the milk is regulated naturally.
7. Breast-fed babies are less prone to eczema, asthma, hay fever and other allergies.
8. Breast feeding produces a hormone which helps the mother's womb to return to its normal size.
9. You and your baby will enjoy the close loving contact.
10. Breast feeding your baby may protect you against breast cancer, as this type of cancer is more common in mothers who do not breast feed.

BREAST IS BEST!

It's safe.
It's free from infection.
It's free.
It's easily accessible –
    anywhere, any time.
It doesn't need warming
The cat can't get at it!
It comes in such lovely
    containers!

BREAST FEEDING

Put your baby to the breast as soon as your baby is born. Not only does this create an immediate strong bond between mother and child, but it can, as reflex action, also help with the delivery of the placenta or afterbirth.

Feed as often as necessary. Every 2 hours is usual for the first couple of days. Although this is very tiring, especially after what may have been an exhausting delivery, try and persevere if you can. The frequent sucking on the breast at this stage can be an investment for the future, as it strongly stimulates the flow of milk.

Give your baby as much breast milk as he will take, but try to equalise the feeding times on each breast. If your baby is hungry he will suckle more voraciously, and this will stimulate a greater supply of milk.

Give only breast milk until the baby is 3 months old, then start introducing solid feeds (see Weaning on page 17).

If possible continue with some breast feeding for as long as you can. The onset of teething with those sharp 'toothy pegs' often brings about a sharp cessation of breast feeding!

If you develop cracked nipples or breast abscesses you may well have to stop breast feeding.

Cracked nipples

These occur as a result of the repeated trauma of constant sucking upon the nipple itself, instead of the nipple and areola (the brown area around the outside of the nipple). It can be very distressing for a mother intent on breast feeding, to have to throw in the towel at this stage.

To prevent this happening, use *Morsep* or *Masse* cream or *Kamillosan ointment* which can be bought over the counter in chemists or can be obtained on prescription from your GP. Rub this cream into the nipples, twice daily, during the last two months of your pregnancy, and then after each breast feed.

Another way to prevent cracked nipples is to make sure that you push the nipple right into the baby's mouth so that he is sucking not just on the nipple but also the areola. If cracked nipples do occur, give breast feeding a rest for 24 hours, express the breast milk into a bottle – your midwife will show the right technique – and give your baby your milk from a bottle. Apply the nipple cream every hour whilst you are not breast feeding, and continue to feed the baby on the other breast if possible.

Breast abscess

This is the result of an infection entering the breast tissue through a cracked nipple in a breast-feeding mother. Part of the breast looks red, feels tender and hard, and you may feel slightly feverish. It lasts from 2 to 10 days. Breast feeding must be stopped, and milk expressed (as above). Good support must be given to the affected breast, whilst you take a course of antibiotics from your doctor. If the abscess does not clear you may have to have the abscess drained at hospital, so to prevent this condition developing, ensure that you prevent cracked nipples and keep your breasts clean by bathing them regularly – especially after feeding.

BOTTLE FEEDING

Feed your newborn as soon as he shows some sort of interest. This commonly occurs within the first 4 hours after delivery.

Your baby will probably settle into a routine of feeding every 3 to 4 hours. If possible feed him when he wants feeding – don't interfere with nature's routines!

How much should you give your baby? Over 24 hours your baby

should receive 2.5 ounces of feed for each pound the baby weighs (2.5 oz/lb). However, don't become too obsessed by this figure, let your baby have what he needs.

Your baby will feed until he is satisfied, and then stop. If your baby is content, happy and growing normally, then he's getting enough from his feeds.

Which bottle feed?

Four types of artificial milk could be given to your baby:

1. Whey-dominant infant formulas.
2. Casein-dominant formulas.
3. Soya-based formulas.
4. Cow's milk.

According to paediatric nutrition experts that's the order of priority, in choosing which feed your baby should receive.

Both whey-dominant and casein-dominant formulas are derived from cow's milk, from which the animal fat has been largely removed and replaced by vegetable fat. Whey-dominant baby milks have had the cow's milk protein modified whereas the casein-dominant baby milks contain unmodified cow's milk protein. So what does all that mean? Basically, you should try the whey-based first and go to casein-based if your baby is not happy with your first choice.

Whey-dominant formulas:
Aptamil from Milupa.
Premium from Cow & Gate.
Ostermilk from Farley's.
SMA Gold from Wyeth.

Casein-dominant formulas:
Milumil from Milupa.
Plus from Cow & Gate.
Ostermilk 2 from Farley's.
SMA White from Wyeth.

Soya-based formulas were introduced for babies who developed an intolerance to the protein content of cow's milk or to the sugar (lactose) present in cow's milk. Such babies cannot tolerate the above-listed popular infant formulas.

Soya-based formulas:
Isomil from Abbott.
Ostersoy from Farley's.
S Formula from Cow & Gate
Sobee from Mead Johnson.
Prosobee from Mead Johnson.
Wysoy from Wyeth.

As mentioned elsewhere, ordinary cow's milk, semi-skimmed milk, skimmed milk, goat's milk etc. are totally unsuitable for babies during their first 12 months.

'DO's AND 'DON'T's OF BOTTLE FEEDING

DO

* Make up only one bottle at a time.

* Only use a pre-sterilised bottle.

* Feed the baby, soon after making up the feed.

* Let him leave some of his feed behind. He's had enough!

* Give him more feed when he empties his bottle. He needs more!

DON'T

* Don't make up 24 hour supplies of feeds. I know it's more convenient, and makes life a lot easier, especially at four in the morning. However, this gives bacteria the time and opportunity to multiply in the milk, even though the milk may be stored in the fridge. Many home refrigerators do not store food at the perfect temperature to inhibit bacterial growth.

* Don't use bottle warmers for the night feed. Any bacteria that may have got into the milk could well grow and incubate at the warm temperature produced by the milk warmer.

* Don't heat feeds in the microwave oven. The outside of the bottle may feel to be just right to the touch but the interior of the bottle and the milk could be much hotter and possible burn the baby's mouth. Remember microwaves heat food and liquids, from the inside outwards.

BABIES AND VITAMIN DROPS

Bottle-fed babies

All infant formulas (powdered baby milks) and follow-on milks are fortified with Vitamins A and D.

Bottle-fed babies receiving standard infant formula baby milks or a follow-on baby milk do NOT therefore need Vitamin drops.

Breast-fed babies

Up to 6 months:

Breast-fed babies under 6 months do NOT need vitamin drops. (For exceptions see below).

The baby will have normally received adequate vitamin supplies from the mother during his growth in her womb.

6 to 12 months:

From 6 MONTHS onwards ALL breast-fed babies should receive vitamin drops.

Five drops per day of Department of Health vitamin drops are needed.

Exceptions

Some breast-fed babies will need these vitamin drops from birth. Vitamin D is needed for strong bone development. It is a very important vitamin to the developing baby as it grows inside the womb. The baby's source of Vitamin D is his mother. Pregnant mothers should ideally receive Vitamin D supplements during pregnancy, but unfortunately very few do! You make Vitamin D yourself when you are exposed to sunshine. If you did not receive Vitamin D during your pregnancy, and you have not had a great deal of exposure to sunlight, you may well have low levels of Vitamin D and your baby may also have low levels of this important vitamin.

The following breast-feeding mothers SHOULD give Vitamin drops to their babies under 6 months of age:

* All Asian mothers.
* All mothers in Northern England, i.e. above the Midlands.
* All mothers who have had a winter pregnancy.

SHOULD I GIVE MY BABY A DUMMY?

Your baby is totally pre-occupied with the four 'S's:

* Sucking.
* Sleeping.
* Soiling nappies.
* Seeing what's going on around him.

16

Sucking is a natural instinctive action which gives him great comfort, even when this activity does not provide him with food!

Imagine the scene:
1. An unhappy screaming baby without a dummy.
2. A silent, contented baby with a dummy.

Forget your principles – what happened to common sense? If you're happy and it satisfies him, let him have a dummy. If you don't he'll suck his thumb or his fingers which can become very sore, or he'll suck his blanket. He'll find something – you decide what you prefer to see him sucking.

WINDING YOUR BABY

While your baby sucks on the bottle or breast he swallows air. It helps to get this air 'up'. We as adults have learnt to burp or belch when necessary. Your baby hasn't learnt that procedure yet, so help him by sitting him upright and gently patting his back. It's the sitting upright that does the trick, not the patting! Wind him twice – once in the middle of his feed and then again at the end. If no wind comes up in the first half minute, get back to feeding him or he will cry and maybe swallow even more air in his distress!

WEANING

As your baby's body grows he obviously will need more nourishment than is supplied by milk alone. Weaning is the introduction of solid foods into the babies daily feeding routine. Bringing solid foods into his diet supplies him with the extra energy, vitamins and minerals he needs to develop normally.

When to introduce solid foods?

Most babies should receive only breast milk or infant formula milk until they are 3 months old. Then start gradually introducing solid foods. All babies should be receiving these as well as their milk by the time they are 6 months old.

What solid foods to introduce?

Cereals

Nearly every baby is weaned onto the cereal-based foods that are widely available commercially. There is a vast selection, and you should enjoy discovering your little baby's likes and dislikes. He will soon progress onto the proper baby meals and some liquidised family foods.

Meat and green vegetables

These are an excellent source of iron, which is necessary to prevent your baby becoming anaemic. Giving your baby vitamin C in the

BABY'S WEIGHT GAIN

* Most babies born at 40 weeks weigh between $5^1/_2$–$9^1/_4$ lbs (2.5–4.2 kg).
* Girls less than $5^1/_2$ lbs (2.5 kg) are classed as small for dates.
* Boys less than $6^1/_2$ lbs (3 kg) are classed as small for dates.
* After delivery your baby will lose a little weight.
* The baby should be back to his birth weight by 10 days.
* Thereafter, usual weight gain is 4–8 ozs (125–250gms)/week. (1 oz = 28.4 gms, 1 gm = 0.035 oz).
* See your GP if baby's weight gain is outside this range.

form of fruit juices along with liquidised green vegetables aids the absorption of iron from those vegetables. If possible give your baby fruit juice from a cup, or spoon, so as to avoid dental caries, which is more prevalent in babies who have been given fruit juice drinks in their baby bottle – the sugar-rich fruit juice is in contact with the teeth for longer in this situation.

Sweets and puddings
These are very tasty to the baby! But they are not a good source of protein. Certainly let you baby have them but do make sure that he has also had his cereals, meat and vegetables beforehand.

Fuller details on weaning can be obtained from your health visitor or local child clinic.

Helpful organisation

National Chilbirth Trust
Alexandra House
Oldham Terrace
London W3 6NH

SLEEPING

We are all different individuals and so our daily requirements of food, exercise, relaxation and sleep vary from person to person. Babies are no different. Some require a lot of sleep and, unfortunately for the poor parents, others don't seem to need much sleep at all! The sleeplessness of the baby does more damage to the parents than it seems to do to the innocent child. Many's the night I've driven around in the car, at four in the morning, with one of our little ones who was intent on an all-night marathon of wakefulness. I discovered that the one thing that induced sleep was to take the little tinker (I'm being rather polite in my choice of language here!) out for a drive. The rhythmic movement of the car was guaranteed to make those eyelids heavy – the child's as well as mine!

AVERAGE HOURS OF SLEEP

BIRTH–1 YEAR

12–18 hours

1–3 YEARS

10–14 hours

3–6 YEARS

9–12 hours

Don't be too upset if your baby doesn't stick to these hours, they are only guidelines - they are NOT rules your baby has to adhere to. Mother Nature is your best guide:

ALL THAT HE SLEEPS IS ALL THAT HE NEEDS!

Babies that do not sleep for long stretches of time are often intelligent, lively and very interested in everything around them. My wife and I had to keep telling ourselves that, night after night. It wasn't a great consolation, when I'd been on call for each of the previous seven nights!

By about the age of 18 months, 70% of babies are sleeping through the whole night.

HOW TO DEAL WITH A CHILD THAT DOES NOT SLEEP:

* Draw up a duty rota, so that one night you're on duty if the baby wakes and the next night your partner is on duty. That way you will be guaranteed 3–4 good nights sleep each week.

* Try to tire your baby out during the day with all sorts of activities and interests – you'll probably shatter yourself in the process, as well!

* As bedtime approaches, don't get the little one too excited. Try to plan a relaxing, winding down routine just before bedtime.

Babies soon come to appreciate a 'set routine', and remember, a routine is a stabilising influence and is very comforting to a young child.

* Soothing music, nursery rhymes, dimmed lighting, cuddling and rocking the child all help to induce a sleepy state of mind. A bedtime feed or drink can be a useful part of the routine. Disconnecting the phone and keeping down the volume on TV, radio and hi-fis can all help, but having said that it's quite surprising how quickly a tired child can sink into a deep sleep despite a cacophony of intense sound blasting out from the teenager's bedroom next door!

* If possible give your baby his own bedroom. A baby that sleeps in your bedroom can disturb your night repeatedly, as you become aware of every breath, groan or sigh that he makes.

* Don't respond immediately when he wakes and cries in the night. Leave him for a while to see if he goes back

to sleep again, and if after 5 to 10 minutes he hasn't done so lift him, straighten his bed, cuddle him, give him a drink or a feed if you think he needs it and maybe he needs a nappy change. Then put him back to bed. Staying with him and sitting by his bed can reassure him enough to help him get back to sleep. Only bring him into *your* bed as a last resort. Babies are not stupid – they are very quick to learn all the tricks in the book! If crying gets him your immediate attention and a full night in the comfort and security of a parent's bed, he'll do it – every night without fail.

* Being hard-hearted and stern does not usually work, it only upsets the child further. So bite your bottom lip firmly and try to remain calm and relaxed – your child is very sensitive to your feelings!

* Leaving a low light on in the baby's bedroom might be helpful.

* Check that his bedding and clothing are not causing any problems. Tight fitting plastic pants or a nappy-pin that's become undone might go unnoticed by a parent, but not by a baby!

* Have plenty of posters on the walls, and plenty of toys and baby books by the bed so that he can amuse himself without disturbing you – fingers crossed!

* If the worst comes to the worst you may have to put up with your baby's erratic sleep patterns. You may end up playing with him when he's awake and sleeping when he sleeps – even if that is during the day! These are the sacrifices you have to make for your children!

Try to be patient. It all works out well in the end – eventually!

If it all does become too much for you, speak to your doctor. He may help by prescribing a short course of a mild sedative to get your child into a sleep routine, and save your sanity.

THE CRYING BABY

WHY IS THE BABY CRYING?

Hunger

Could he be hungry?
When was he last fed?
Was the last feed smaller than his usual feed?
Has he been sick since the last feed?
Is he having enough to eat?
Should he be on more than just milk?

Action

Feed him (see page 10).

Thirst

Is he thirsty?
Is it warm weather?
Is the room very warm?
Does the baby look hot, i.e. flushed?
Is his temperature raised?

Action

Cool him, cool the room.
Give him drinks.
Use a thermometer to take his temperature.

Pain

Is he screaming?
Is he restless?
Is he distressed?
Is he pulling on his ears?
Is he pulling up his legs?
Is he screaming when passing water (urine)?
Has he fallen or injured himself?
Is he teething? (There is some controversy about this causing pain in a baby)

Action

Contact GP, describing in full what is happening to your baby.

Illness

Is he feverish?
Is there a rash anywhere on his body?
Is he off his food?
Is he crying whilst being fed?
- Possible throat infection
Are there any white spots on his tongue and inside his cheeks? (Probably thrush)
Has he got diarrhoea?
Is he vomiting?
Is his nose runny?
Is he coughing?
Is he having breathing difficulty?
Is he wheezing?
Have his lips or fingers turned blue?
Is there any blood in his urine?
Is there any blood in his stools?
Has he become pale?

Does his cry sound unusual?
Has he lost interest in his
surroundings?
Is he drowsy, so that you
cannot rouse him?
Has he become limp or
floppy?

Action
Contact GP immediately.

———

Unhappy
Is his nappy wet or dirty?
Is he bored or lonely?
Is he tired? - Has he missed a
nap?

Action
Change nappy.
Play with him – sit him
upright and let him see

what's going on around
him.
Cuddle him and rock him to
sleep.

———

Personality
Some babies just cry a lot.

Two of our four children were very
trying! They cried a great deal, for
no obvious reason, and they always
seemed to cry more at night!

If everything is getting too much
for you and you feel that you are at
the end of your tether because of
the incessant crying, do get in
contact with your GP, health visitor,
practice nurse, midwife or local
clinic. Health professionals are
there to help you – use them!

23

NAPPY RASH

What is nappy rash?

Nappy rash is very, very common. Most babies will have nappy rash at some time during their development.

What you see is:
* A redness in the skin around the genitals and anal area. This redness may spread to the rest of the skin covered by the nappy, from the navel down to the thighs.
* Infected yellow spots may develop.
* Skin may flake off leaving raw red areas, which are very tender.

Who gets nappy rash?

Any baby – though it occurs more commonly in babies who are bottle fed, and in babies who are left for long periods of time in their wet nappy. Babies who have diabetes, eczema and loose stools are also more prone to it.

What causes nappy rash?

The commonest causes of nappy rash are:

* Ammonia
* Thrush
* Detergents.

Ammonia: Ammonia is a very strong chemical which when in contact with skin, causes a mild 'burn' to the superficial skin layers. So how does your baby come into contact with ammonia?
In a baby's stools or faeces (*fee-sees*), there are bacteria which when in contact with the baby's urine cause a breakdown of the urine to produce the chemical – ammonia. If that ammonia is in contact with the skin for too long it actually creates a chemical burn to the skin! Sounds horrific doesn't it? But that's just what a severe nappy rash looks like – a burn! The skin is very sore and tender, and the baby is very, very uncomfortable – especially when further ammonia comes into contact with the raw skin which, if you are using non-disposable nappies, is then rubbed repeatedly by towelling material!

Thrush: Thrush is quite a common infection in babies. If the baby has a thrush infection of the mouth, the organism passes down through the baby's intestines and out in the baby's stools. The infection is caused by a fungus, candida, and this grows like any other fungus, where the conditions of dampness, darkness and warmth prevail. Underneath a wet nappy, inside the plastic pants is absolute heaven for the thrush fungus! When the word fungus is mentioned, pictures of mushrooms come straight to mind – no, you *don't* get mushrooms growing on the skin!

What you do see is a red rash affecting the skin in the nappy area, which is itchy and tender. At the edges of the red areas you will see discrete little red spots spreading onto normal skin. These are known as satellite lesions and are one of the classical signs of an infection of the skin caused by thrush.

Detergents: Detergents and biological washing powders are strong chemicals. All babies have sensitive skins that can react quite severely when in contact with these irritant chemicals.

The rash produced by these substances is called a 'contact dermatitis', and as with other types of nappy rash the skin is red, inflamed and tender. Often tiny little blisters appear on the skin with a contact dermatitis, and in some cases this 'detergent' rash can even be superimposed upon a nappy rash caused by ammonia or thrush!

Can you prevent nappy rash?
Yes it certainly can be prevented – as always prevention is the best form of treatment (see page 26).

10-POINT PLAN FOR A BEAUTIFUL BOTTOM!

1. Try to breast feed your baby. Nappy rash is less common in breast-fed babies.

2. After removing the wet or dirty nappy, gently clean the skin with either warm water, or cotton wool and baby lotion/baby oil, or special baby-cleaning tissues. Dry gently and *thoroughly*.

3. Apply liberal amounts of a barrier cream, such as zinc and castor oil, which acts as a waterproof barrier preventing skin contact with urine and stools. There's no need to use talcum powder, it forms clumps in the skin folds, which can cause skin reactions.

4. If you use towelling nappies, always ensure that they are thoroughly rinsed out in clear water after washing, and thoroughly aired. Avoid using biological or strong detergents, use gentle soap flakes instead.

25

5. The nappy rash due to ammonia can be prevented by rinsing towelling nappies in water containing vinegar. Ammonia is alkaline which can be neutralised by adding an acid to it. Vinegar is mildly acidic – it is acetic acid. Put two tablespoons of vinegar into every one gallon of water – do the final rinse in this water, then hang the nappies out to dry.

6. Change your baby's nappy frequently. Never allow him to lie for long in a wet or dirty nappy.

7. When possible leave the nappy off, to allow fresh air to circulate over the skin. At this point you can guarantee that little boys will send a stream of urine cascading over the pram, carpet, cot or themselves! Whereas, little girls just do it where they're lying!

8. Don't use tight-fitting plastic pants. Urine should ideally be allowed to evaporate from a wet nappy, through looser fitting pants. If your baby is prone to repeated episodes of nappy rash then you may have to consider avoiding the routine use of plastic pants.

9. Using disposable nappies and one-way disposable nappy liners, makes life a lot easier, and can help a great deal to prevent nappy rash. But there is a cost element to consider, as well as an environmental issue (trees used for paper, disposal problems, etc.).

10. Prompt treatment of oral thrush will help to prevent the condition from spreading to the nappy area.

How do you treat nappy rash? Yourself:

Barrier creams that are effective in preventing and treating nappy rash and which you can buy from your local pharmacy are:

Kamillosan ointment.
Morhulin ointment.
Morsep cream.
Rikospray Silicone aerosol.
Siopel cream.
Sudocrem cream.
Thovaline aerosol and ointment.
Unguentum cream.
Zinc and castor oil cream.

Changing to a different brand of disposable nappy might improve things, or even changing to towelling.

GP:

If the above measures do not work, take your baby to see your GP. If the doctor diagnoses thrush as the cause of your baby's nappy rash, you will be prescribed an anti-fungal cream to apply to the bottom.

The most popular anti-thrush creams are:

Nystatin
Nystaform
Nystan

Apply these three times a day until one week after the skin has cleared. Other anti-fungal creams sometimes used are *Canesten* and *Daktarin*.

An antibiotic cream may be prescribed if a bacterial infection has been superimposed upon the nappy rash.

Nappy rashes are not serious, although they can look quite shocking and repulsive. They are easily treated and usually do respond very quickly to treatment.

COT DEATH

What is cot death?
Cot death, also known as Sudden Infant Death Syndrome (SIDS), is defined as 'the sudden death of any infant or young child which is unexplained and in which a thorough postmortem examination fails to demonstrate an adequate cause of death'.

It is the commonest presentation of death for children aged 1 week to 2 years. Having said that, the condition itself is rare in the community, occurring in 1 in 500 live births. An average GP will see only one every 10 years.

It is extremely difficult to come to terms with, as no obvious reason can be given for the child's death. Every parent has been worried at some time about their own child becoming a victim of this distressing condition.

The commonest story is that a deeply shocked parent just finds their baby dead in the cot, without any obvious prior warning or indication that anything was wrong with the child.

Who develops cot death?
It occurs most commonly between the ages of 1 month and 6 months,

with a peak incidence in 2 and 3 month-old babies. Before discussing the latest evidence that shows when cot death seems to occur most frequently, I just want to say something to those parents who have suffered the tragedy of a cot death.

'When you read what follows, you may feel terrible guilt in that, had you not laid your baby a certain way, or had you not put so much bedding on the baby, maybe your baby might still be with you today.

The evidence is confusing and bewildering. We do not know any single cause of cot death. My writings are based on the latest medical research which you could not have known about at the time.

According to today's latest medical knowledge I myself, a doctor, and my wife, a midwifery sister, obviously did the wrong things with our own young babies – but we were lucky. Without access to up-to-date medical findings, no one could know what factors predispose little babies to this sudden loss of life.

If this item on cot death provides you and other readers with the knowledge to avoid certain risks affecting your next infant, then it will have been well worth it, for now that you are armed with this latest information you can be reassured that you are doing your utmost to prevent this tragedy.'

Cot death occurs more commonly in the following situations:

* In babies born prematurely.
* In babies laid in bed in the face-down position.
* In babies who have become overheated, e.g. heating left on in the bedroom all night, excessive bedding on the baby, or wrapping babies too tightly in their bedding.

Other factors that can predispose a baby to cot death are shown by the fact that cot death is more common in:

* Baby boys.
* Babies born in the winter months.
* Babies born of single parents.
* Babies born of mothers who had little ante-natal care.
* Babies born of smoking mothers.
* Babies who are bottle-fed.
* Babies with congenital abnormalities.
* Babies born as triplets.
* Babies who have brothers and sisters.
* Babies with low birth-weight.

* Babies who were unwell on the day before death.
* Babies of drug-abusing mothers.

Research is also looking at the possibility that certain viral chest infections may be implicated, and also that old PVC mattresses may give off toxic gases that could have an effect upon the baby.

What is the cause of cot death?

There is no known single cause of this condition. As you can see from the section above, there seem to be many different factors which may be influential. There is extensive research going on at present to try to define the factors which have such devastating effects upon a young baby.

Can you prevent cot death?

On looking through the list of factors common to a number of cot deaths (as above) you will see that certain situations or risk are avoidable. In reducing the risks, think:

* BED
* BEDROOM
* BEDDING

and think

* NOT HOT

COT DEATH – REDUCING THE RISKS

BED: When putting your baby to bed, lay your baby FACE UP.

BEDROOM: The bedroom must NOT be HOT.
  – do NOT have the heating on all night.
  – keep the bedroom COOL, neither cold nor hot – COOL.

BEDDING: The bedding must NOT be too HOT or too tight.
  – rather than a duvet, use a sheet and 2 or 3 blankets. If your baby feels hot remove some of the covers.
  – keep the bedding loose, so that he can kick the blankets off if he is getting too hot.

Follow these instructions:

EVEN IN WINTER
EVEN IF YOUR BABY HAS A TEMPERATURE

After the age of 1 month, babies in the modern home, do NOT need more clothing than adults.

COT DEATH PARENTS

For parents who have suffered the loss of their baby through cot death, I would strongly recommend that you do not rush into another pregnancy. A one-year gap is suggested, as it will take the family at least that length of time to partially overcome their distress, and it is also mentally and physically exhausting to have a pregnancy so soon after another. In any subsequent pregnancy, you should receive good support throughout from your ante-natal clinic, midwife, GP, and health visitor until the child is 1 year old.

Apnoea (*app-neeyah*) monitors that are connected to the baby when he is put down to sleep, and sound an alarm if he stops breathing are very reassuring items. Parents can then adopt a near normal lifestyle without having obsessively to watch over their little one. These monitors may be provided from your local hospital.

Apnoea monitors are available from:
Eastleigh Alarms
(NH Eastwood Ltd)
118 East Barnet Road
Barnet
Herts EN4 8RE

Helpful organisation
I can strongly recommend that the following organisations be contacted:

The Foundation for the Study of Infant Deaths,
15 Belgrave Square,
London SW1X 8PS
Helpline: 071-235-1721

CONI (Care of the Next Infant),
Room C1,
Stephenson Unit,
Sheffield Children's Hospital,
University of Sheffield,
Western Bank,
Sheffield S10 2TH.

IMMUNISATION

Immunisation protects your child against diseases that can kill. Immunisation works and is simple and safe. Although some of the infectious diseases are quite common, we must realise that these diseases can be very serious, and there is no room for complacency.

Childhood diseases
can be serious.

They can strike

ANY CHILD –
ANYWHERE – ANY TIME

Childhood infectious diseases can have disastrous results on the affected child:

* Blindness
* Deafness
* Paralysis
* Brain Damage
* Death

Measles can cause encephalitis (inflammation of the brain), which often results in permanent damage to the brain. Other consequences of measles are pneumonia, bronchitis and deafness from ear infections.

Whooping cough produces difficulty in breathing, vomiting, weight loss and extremely distressing long bouts of coughing. Lung damage, convulsions and even death have resulted from whooping cough.

The risk of any serious complications from immunisation is far LESS than the risks your child will face from getting the actual diseases themselves.

Serious **PREVENTABLE** childhood diseases are:

Diphtheria (*diff-thee-ree-ah*)
Tetanus
Whooping cough (Pertussis)
Polio
Measles
Mumps
Rubella (*roo-bella*) or German measles

31

As a result of effective immunisation programmes, smallpox has been totally eradicated worldwide since 1971. Through effective vaccination programmes, the UK Department of Health is aiming to eradicate totally all children's infectious diseases by the year 2000. This elimination process is starting to happen – immunisation rates are at record levels and the number of children catching measles, whooping cough and mumps is declining. Polio is now rarely seen.

How does immunisation work?
Immunisation works by subjecting your body to a very mild or altered form of the organism, be it virus or bacteria, that causes the disease. When your child receives this form of the disease through an injection the only adverse effect is a slight soreness at the injection site, with a possibility of slight fever and feeling a little unwell for 12 to 24 hours afterwards. Many children have no adverse effects whatsoever.

When your child is immunised with the organism, the body's defences come into play and produce antibodies to attack and destroy the invading organism. This stimulation of antibody production gives your child long-term protection against that disease. Whenever your child comes into contact with that virus or bacteria

IMMUNISATION TIMETABLE

Age	Disease	Method
2 mths	Diphtheria, Whooping Cough, Tetanus	– one injection
	Polio	– orally
3 mths	Diphtheria, Whooping Cough, Tetanus	– one injection
	Polio	– orally
4 mths	Diphtheria, Whooping Cough, Tetanus	– one injection
	Polio	– orally
12–18 mths	Measles, Mumps, Rubella (MMR)	– one injection
4–5 yrs	Diphtheria, Tetanus	– one injection
	Polio	– orally
10–13 yrs	Rubella (for girls who did NOT receive the MMR vaccine when younger)	– one injection
13 yrs	Tuberculosis (BCG)	– one injection
16 yrs	Tetanus	– one injection
	Polio	– orally

he will have the ability to attack and kill the organisms with his own antibodies. Your child will have developed long-lasting resistance to that disease as a result of being immunised.

It makes sense to have your child immunised!

Notes
The young adult reaching 16 years of age now has protection from diphtheria, tetanus, whooping cough, polio, measles, mumps, rubella and tuberculosis.

Boosters for polio and tetanus are recommended every 10 years. No boosters are recommended for the other diseases.

WRONG REASONS FOR NOT VACCINATING
False beliefs are held by many parents and even some members of the medical profession about who should and who should not be vaccinated.

Children in the following groups SHOULD BE IMMUNISED!

* Children with asthma, eczema or allergies.
* Children with a family history of asthma, eczema or allergies.

* Children who are 'chesty' or 'snuffly' on the day of their injections, but otherwise well.
* Children on antibiotics.
* Children on steroid creams or steroid inhalers.
* Children with a family history of convulsions in relatives more distant than parents, brothers or sisters.
* Children with congenital heart disease.
* Children with chronic lung disease.
* Children who were born premature, or of low birth-weight.
* Children with Down's syndrome or other chromosome disorder.
* Children with cerebral palsy.
* Children being breast-fed.
* Children whose mothers are again pregnant.

THE VACCINES
There used to be only one 'triple' vaccine – diphtheria, pertussis (whooping cough) and tetanus – known as DPT.

A second 'triple' vaccine is now given to children – measles, mumps and rubella (German measles). This is known as the MMR vaccine. It is now better to forget the term

33

> ## IF MY CHILD HAS ALREADY HAD ONE OF THE INFECTIOUS DISEASES SHOULD HE BE VACCINATED?
>
> Even if your child has had measles, mumps or rubella, it is still best to receive the MMR vaccine.

'triple' vaccine and just call them the DPT and MMR vaccines.

Diphtheria
Combined with tetanus and whooping cough into one single injection. Side effects are uncommon and usually not troublesome. Slight irritability and slight fever may occur 12–24 hours after the injection. The injection site may show a slight swelling or reddening. If there is a more marked reaction contact your doctor for further advice. Children over 10 years, and adults who are receiving this vaccine for the first time, can have a more severe reaction at the injection site and should therefore be given a special low-dose adsorbed diphtheria vaccine for adults.

Whooping cough
Also known as pertussis. Combined with diphtheria and tetanus in one single injection. A great deal of concern has arisen from the possibility of an association between brain damage and whooping cough vaccine. After close examination of all the research relating to this controversial issue, the Department of Health has concluded that it is safer for your child to receive the vaccine than to chance catching the disease with all its associated serious complications. Evidence from extensive research into this area has shown that:

* there is NO convincing argument that the whooping cough vaccine results in permanent brain or nerve damage.

* whooping cough vaccine does NOT cause epilepsy.

* there is NO convincing evidence of a link between the vaccine and cot death (Sudden Infant Death Syndrome).

* there is NO convincing evidence that children with a history of neurological disease (disorders of the

brain or nervous system) or a family history of convulsions, will deteriorate more rapidly if they receive the vaccine, although a paediatrician should be consulted on this matter.

* possible brain damage as a result of the whooping cough vaccine is so rare that a GP with an average patient list size would only see this once in 1,500 years! This should hopefully put it into some sort of perspective. All my four children received the whooping cough vaccine!

THE VACCINE IS SAFE
–
THE DISEASE IS
DANGEROUS

Tetanus
Combined with diphtheria and whooping cough and given as an injection. No serious side effects. Booster should be given every 10 years to maintain high immunity. Unlike today's children, parents born before 1961 will not have received a routine course of tetanus. Check with your doctor for advice.

Polio
A live virus vaccine given by drops into the mouth. Mild reactions such as slight fever or very mild swelling of glands in the neck rarely occur. Parents born before 1958, may not have received routine polio immunisation, and you may find that your doctor is keen to give the oral polio drops at the same time as your child.

Measles
Combined with mumps and rubella (German measles) in the MMR vaccine, it can cause minor symptoms such as fever and a mild rash usually between 5 to 10 days after vaccination.

Mumps
Combined with measles and rubella in the MMR vaccine. Side effects are uncommon. After 3–4 weeks 1 child in 100 might develop slight swelling at the side of the face in front of the ear – a mild form of one-sided mumps!

Rubella (German measles)
Combined with measles and mumps in the MMR vaccine. Although rubella is a mild, non-serious disease in itself, children are vaccinated against it to prevent its occurrence later in life in women during pregnancy. If a woman has not been vaccinated against rubella,

and subsequently develops rubella in early pregnancy, the disease can severely affect her unborn child. The baby could be blind, deaf, have severe abnormalities of the heart or could be mentally retarded. The vaccination is safe and there are no troublesome side effects. A pregnant mum who has never had rubella is quite safe to come into contact with a child who has received the rubella vaccine.

WHEN SHOULD VACCINES *NOT* BE GIVEN?

If your child is ill or has a fever of over 38°C postpone the vaccination to another date.

Specific vaccines should NOT be given to children in the following circumstances:

POLIO: If the child has active diarrhoea.

MEASLES: Only if the child has had a severe (anaphylactic) reaction to eggs or egg products.

Children who have convulsions (fits), or whose parents or brothers and sisters have had epilepsy MUST BE IMMUNISED. Fits brought on by high temperatures can be prevented by prompt treatment with paracetamol. In the USA these children are given their immunisation and are treated with paracetamol for 2–3 days. Paracetamol should also be handy for these children about a week after the vaccine, as the feverish reaction can occur between the 7th and 10th day after immunisation.

MMR: As for measles.

WHOOPING COUGH: The only reason for a child NOT to receive this vaccine is that the child suffered a severe reaction to a previous dose.

A severe reaction is defined as:

* Extensive redness, swelling and hardening of the injected limb and/or

* A fever over 39.5°C, within 48 hours and/or

* Severe allergic reaction (anaphylaxis), collapse, difficulty in breathing, prolonged screaming or convulsions within 72 hours.

FINAL WORD
These common diseases can kill. All my four children have been fully vaccinated, so come on Mums

IMMUNISATION RECORD			
Vaccine	Age Due	Name	Date Given
1st DTP & Polio	2 mths		
2nd DTP & Polio	3 mths		
3rd DTP & Polio	4 mths		
MMR	12-18 mths		
Diptheria/ Tetanus & Polio (Booster)	4-5 yrs		
Rubella (girls) if MMR not given	10–13 yrs		
Tuberculosis (BCG)	13 yrs		
Tetanus and Polio (Booster)	15 yrs		

and Dads, let's get rid of all these infectious diseases once and for all. It can be done, we've already done it with smallpox. Take your children down to your GP's surgery or to your local children's clinic, and keep a record of their immunisations on the table on page 37, or you may prefer to photocopy it and keep it with other medical records.

REMEMBER
THE INJECTION
IS SAFER THAN
THE INFECTION!

Information on these infectious diseases and their management can be found in the next chapter.

Helpful organisation
For further information contact your local Health Promotion Unit, their address or telephone number can be obtained from your GP or local hospital.

You can also get information directly from:

The Health Education Authority
Hamilton House
Mabledon Place
London WC1H 9TX

INFECTIOUS DISEASES

THE INFECTIOUS DISEASES

The common infectious children's diseases can be divided into two categories 'spotty' and 'non-spotty':

Spotty
  Measles
  Rubella (German measles)
  Chickenpox
  Scarlet fever

Non-spotty
  Whooping cough
  Mumps

As all infectious diseases are more severe when they occur in adults, people argue that it is better to get these infections as a child. In fact, it is NOT better to catch these infections as a child, it is unwise to get them AT ANY AGE, as they are potentially serious diseases. We can all be fully protected by vaccination.

Get
INJECTED
–
Not
INFECTED!

DISAPPEARING DISEASES!

Other infectious diseases (all 'non-spotty'), which your child will have been vaccinated against, are:

Diphtheria
Tetanus
Polio
Tuberculosis (TB)

Fortunately, these four diseases which used to kill and cripple our children in the past, are now rare in the western world as a direct result of active immunisation programmes.

THERE'S A RASH – WHAT'S THE DISEASE?

The Clues

	Before the rash	The rash
Scarlet Fever	Child is ill, with SORE THROAT and HIGH fever	Red rash Lasts 4–5 days
Measles	Child is ill, with RUNNY NOSE, SORE EYES, COUGHING and HIGH fever	Red rash Lasts 4–5 days
Chickenpox	Child may have SLIGHT fever	Tiny blisters that itch and turn to scabs Last 7–10 days
Rubella	May have SLIGHT fever	Pale pink rash Lasts 2–3 days

CHICKENPOX

What is chickenpox?

Chickenpox is another common infectious disease caused by a virus.

Before the spots

After an incubation period of 17–21 days, there may be a slight fever with mild headache, most patients have no symptoms at all until the spots appear.

The spots

The spots of chickenpox can be very itchy. They appear:

First – on the head and trunk. Next – on the arms and legs. They last for 7–10 days.

The spots look like tiny blisters on a red base. They can occur wherever there is skin, even in the mouth, inside the eyelids, up the nose, inside the ears, inside the vagina and inside the anus (back passage). Itchy spots in awkward places can be very distressing to the child. The blisters dry and crust over, and are infectious until the crusts have dropped off. The spots of chickenpox can cause shallow scars. This occurs if some of the spots become infected or have been scratched badly during their itchy phase.

To reduce this risk of scarring see *How should you treat chickenpox?* in the next column.

Complications:
Chickenpox is usually not serious. Only rarely may there be complications such as encephalitis. There may be a risk to the unborn baby if a pregnant mother develops the disease, or to the newborn baby if mother develops chickenpox within 5 days of delivery.

What causes chickenpox?
The virus that causes chickenpox is a member of the herpes virus family. This family of viruses is implicated in cold sores, shingles and genital herpes.

Can you prevent chickenpox?
There is, currently, no vaccination against chickenpox, although research in this area looks promising. Little can be done to prevent your child getting this disease and as it is not a serious disease, your child is better to get this condition 'over and done with' before adulthood. Adults certainly do have a terrible time when they catch chickenpox! The little

blisters of chickenpox are full of liquid containing the virus so the spots are highly infectious. So if Mum or Dad have not had chickenpox, don't touch the spots, and don't use your child's towel!

How should you treat chickenpox?
Yourself:
* Keep child cool – cool room, cool drinks, cool bed.
* Paracetamol may ease pain of spots in sensitive areas.
* Calamine lotion applied to skin can relieve itchiness.
* Leave nappies off to allow spots to dry.

INCUBATION PERIODS
The time between contact and appearance of symptoms

Scarlet Fever
1–5 days

Measles
7 – 14 days

Whooping Cough
7–14 days

Mumps
12–21 days

Chickenpox
14–21 days

Rubella (German measles)
14–21 days

* Keep child's fingernails short.
* Keep off school until crusts have come off spots.

GP:
* Contact GP to confirm diagnosis.
* Call GP:
  – if child is very distressed.
  – if spots show presence of pus.
  – if child is feverish.
  – if child has neckache or severe headache.
  – if you are worried!

Helpful organisation
Information is available from the Health Education Authority (for address see page 38)

MEASLES

What is measles?
Measles is a highly infectious, common disease that is potentially dangerous. Measles is like a 'heavy cold with a rash!'. The child looks miserable with a runny nose, sore eyes and a cough. A red rash follows and spreads all over the body - no wonder it's often called "MISERABLE MEASLES". Measles makes the child unwell even before the rash appears.

Before the rash:
The commonest symptoms to appear are:

* Cough.
* Runny nose.
* Red, runny, sore eyes.
* High temperature – up to 40°C.
* Headache.

All these last for 3–5 days

Your doctor may look inside your child's mouth to check for grey-white specks on the inside of the cheeks. These are called Koplik's spots which only occur in measles.

The rash
After 3 to 5 days of cold-like symptoms, the rash appears:

First - behind the ears and on the neck.
Next - onto the trunk, the arms and then the legs.
They last for 4 to 5 days.

Once the rash has appeared you may then be able to work out who your child was in contact with about 2 weeks ago. Amongst those friends there will probably be one or more who has come down with measles!

The skin looks blotchy and the spots vary from pink to dark red.

The blotches often merge to form a large red mass. The spots do not usually itch. Pale brown staining of the skin occurs as the rash fades. This staining disappears over the next ten days.

Complications

1 in every 15 children with measles will suffer a complication such as deafness, bronchitis, pneumonia, convulsions or even encephalitis (inflammation of the brain).

These are serious problems, which can easily be avoided by having your child immunised with MMR vaccine (see page 33).

Who gets measles?

Anyone who has not had measles or who hasn't been vaccinated and has been in contact with someone who actually has the disease or is incubating the disease. A child incubating the disease may appear well or may just appear to have a cough or a cold, because they have not YET developed the obvious measles rash.

What causes measles?

Measles is caused by a type of virus called a myxovirus. The virus is spread in tiny droplets of saliva from an infected child when they cough or sneeze – even before they have the rash! 10–14 days after being in contact with an infectious child the symptoms may start to appear.

Can you prevent measles?

The only effective way to prevent your child from catching measles is to get him immunised (see chapter on Immunisation on page 31).

FACTS

50% of the children who die as a result of measles are healthy children who have NOT been vaccinated.

Measles is RARE under the age of 9 months because the baby receives protection from Mum's antibodies.

How should you treat measles?

Yourself:
* Keep temperature down.
* Cool room, cool sponge, cool drinks, cool bed.
* Give paracetamol syrup.
* Give plenty of fluids, frequently.

GP:
* Contact GP to confirm diagnosis.

43

* Call GP
  – if fever does not respond.
  – if earache develops.
  – if cough worsens.
  – if fits or drowsiness
    develop.
  – if worried at all!

An antibiotic may be prescribed for a chest infection or an ear infection. The antibiotic does not clear up the measles. There is no cure for measles, it will clear up on its own.

RUBELLA

What is rubella?

Rubella, also known as German measles, is a mild illness that causes very few problems to the sufferer. It is so mild and short-lived that it is notoriously difficult to diagnose.

Its incubation period is 2–3 weeks. There may be a slight runny nose with mild swelling of glands at the back of the neck and behind the ears. This may be followed by a pale pink rash that spreads from the face onto the trunk. This faint rash may last for 2–3 days. The patient rarely has a fever. Adults may experience aching in the joints.

Who gets rubella?

Any unvaccinated person who has been in contact with someone

RUBELLA IN PREGNANCY

Many people have had rubella without knowing a thing about it. An unvaccinated adult may actually have the disease, without realising, and come into contact with a woman in early pregnancy who has not had rubella or the vaccination. That unvaccinated woman may not even know that she is in very early pregnancy!

If that woman, in her early pregnancy, picks up the virus severe abnormalities can develop in her unborn baby. If she is less than 10 weeks pregnant there is a 90% likelihood of her baby being malformed. Babies affected can suffer from deafness, blindness, severe abnormalities of the heart and mental retardation.

Rubella does not affect adults – it deforms unborn babies. Make sure YOUR daughter receives the MMR vaccine in order to protect HER children from these dreadful effects.

either suffering from the disease, or incubating the disease.

What causes rubella?

Rubella is caused by a virus, that is spread in a similar fashion to the measles virus – droplets spread from an infected person. As the old saying goes, "Coughs and sneezes spread diseases".

Can you prevent rubella?

Simple – by immunisation with the MMR vaccine (see page 33).

How should you treat rubella?

Special treatment is rarely needed. Give the child plenty of fluids and keep any temperature under control. Keep the child away from any woman known to be in early pregnancy. A pregnant woman coming into contact with a case of rubella should consult her GP.

Helpful organisation

Information is available from the Health Education Authority (for address see page 38).

WHOOPING COUGH

What is whooping cough?

Whooping cough is also known as pertussis. It is a highly infectious disease which can be very dangerous in the first year of life.

After an incubation period of 7–14 days, the child begins with what appears to be an ordinary cold and a cough. The child develops:

* A fever.
* A runny nose.
* A cough which, after about 10 days, becomes very severe and frightening for the child.

The whoop: the child experiences bouts of coughing which are so persistent that breathing in becomes difficult. After continual coughing the child attempts to gasp for air and as the air is inhaled down through the inflamed airways a peculiar whooping sound is produced. Once heard, this sound is never forgotten! Whooping cough is an horrendous experience for the child, the parents and the family. Throughout the night the poor child coughs, coughs, coughs, whoops as he fights for breath, then coughs, coughs and coughs again, followed by more gasping for breath and whooping. The unrelenting session finally ends with the child vomiting. This coughing phase can last for two months. The child becomes exhausted. The strain of coughing can burst blood vessels in the eye turning the white part of the eye bright red. A child with whooping cough is a sorry sight!

45

This disease can be serious in babies. Inability to breathe in after a coughing spasm can turn the child blue and has proven fatal in some cases. The immense strain of coughing can damage the sensitive lungs and cause blood vessels in the brain to rupture to produce a brain haemorrhage. Vomiting can lead to dehydration, and further problems include convulsions, ear infections and lung infections such as bronchopneumonia and bronchiolitis.

Who gets whooping cough?

Any child that has not been vaccinated is at high risk of picking up this dangerous disease. Despite all the controversy about side effects from the vaccine, I strongly recommend immunisation against this disease – the first injection to be given at the age of 2 months (see the chapter on Immunisation on page 31 for more information).

What causes whooping cough?

Unlike many of the infectious diseases, whooping cough is not caused by a virus but by another type of infecting organism – a bacterium. This 'bug' or bacterium is spread through minute droplets that are propelled through the air when the child coughs or sneezes. The disease is very infectious.

Can you prevent whooping cough?

There is only one way to prevent this disease from affecting your child – immunisation at 2 months, 3 months and 4 months! This disease can be eradicated.

How should you treat whooping cough?

Yourself:
* Keep temperature down (see Fever Control on page 50).
* During a coughing spasm sit your child upright, holding a bowl under the chin for him to cough any sputum or vomit into.
* If possible sleep in the same room. Coughing bouts, gasping for air and vomiting can be frightening for a child alone at night.
* During the day give him drinks and small snacks immediately after a coughing bout that ends in vomiting. You have to get some nourishment into him before the next coughing spasm starts.
* DO NOT SMOKE near your child.

The cough can persist for 8–12 weeks, so do be patient!

GP:
IF YOU SUSPECT WHOOPING COUGH, CONTACT YOUR GP IMMEDIATELY

Little babies rarely whoop. So if your baby has a cold followed by a cough that is worsening, contact your GP. He may take special swabs to confirm the diagnosis. If given early in the course of the disease certain antibiotics, such as erythromycin and cotrimoxazole, can modify the attack.

Your GP may prescribe sedation, such as *Vallergan* or *Phenergan*, for night-time use, but sedatives and cough medicines have not been proven to be of any great benefit.

SCARLET FEVER

What is scarlet fever?
Basically, scarlet fever (also known as scarlatina) is a sore throat with a widespread red rash.

Before the rash
The child has:
* a sore throat.
* infected tonsils.
* furred tongue with tiny red spots.
* a high temperature.
* vomiting and sometimes tummy pains.

The rash of scarlet fever spreads all over the body but is often absent from around the mouth. This white area is known as 'circumoral pallor'.

The rash
Within 3 days the 'lobster-red' rash of scarlet fever appears:

First – on chest and back
Next – spreading to the rest of the body.
It lasts 4–5 days.

The skin often flakes after the rash has gone.

Complications
These are rare, but sometimes nephritis (kidney inflammation) or rheumatic fever (inflammation of the joints and heart valves) occurs.

Who gets scarlet fever?
Anyone could get this condition, but it is rare nowadays and seldom serious.

What causes scarlet fever?
This disease is caused by a bacterium called streptococcus that causes sore throats and tonsillitis.

A toxin is produced by this bacterium which causes the rash and complications of scarlet fever. Antibiotics have now reduced this condition to a rare and mild disease.

Can you prevent scarlet fever?
This disease is not one to be feared and so there is no vaccine.

How should you treat scarlet fever?
Yourself:
* Keep your child at home.
* Keep temperature down (see Fever Control on page 50), bed rest is not essential.
* You should check
  – has child got a fever?
  – has child got swollen, red tonsils?
  – has child got furred tongue with red patches?

If YES to any of above call your GP.

GP:
Will prescribe antibiotics, such as penicillin or erythromycin.

MUMPS

What is mumps?
Mumps, in children, is usually a mild infectious disease, classically producing swellings at the side of the face. These swellings are due to enlargement and inflammation of the glands that produce saliva. The affected glands lie just below and just in front of the ears. They are called the parotid glands.

There is NO RASH with mumps.

After a long incubation period of 3 weeks these symptoms appear:

* Child may feel unwell for a day or two.
* Swelling of the face develops – on one or both sides.
* The swollen glands are often painful.
* Swallowing may be uncomfortable.
* Dry mouth: the inflamed glands produce less saliva.
* Headache and fever.

Complications
Orchitis in boys. This is inflammation of the testes. It is a painful condition, often affecting only one testis which becomes swollen and tender. Even if both testes are affected sterility (inability to have children on reaching adulthood) is exceptionally rare.

Other uncommon side effects of mumps are:

* Deafness

* Pancreatitis – causing upper abdominal pain.
* Meningitis
* Encephalitis (inflammation of the brain)
* Mastitis (inflammation of breasts)
* Oophoritis (inflammation of ovaries)

Who gets mumps?

Any person who has not had mumps before or who has not been vaccinated.

What causes mumps?

It is caused by a virus that enters the body through the mouth or nose. Droplet spread from an infected person is the normal mode of transmission. Patients are infectious until the swollen glands decrease in size.

Can mumps be prevented?

Although the complications of mumps are rare, they are so serious, e.g. meningitis and encephalitis, that avoidance of this disease is

---

HOW LONG IS YOUR CHILD INFECTIOUS?

'Spotty'

CHICKENPOX
Infectious till ALL spots have scabbed over

MEASLES, RUBELLA and SCARLET FEVER
Infectious till 4 days after onset of rash

'Non-spotty'

MUMPS
Infectious till 7 days after swellings have cleared

WHOOPING COUGH
Infectious till 4–6 WEEKS after the onset of the symptoms

extremely necessary. A single injection of the MMR vaccine between 12–18 months gives full protection against mumps. As the Health Education Authority adverts say:

"Give your child something you never had – the MMR vaccine."

How should you treat mumps?
Yourself:
* Control fever (see Fever Control below).
* Give soups and liquidised foods.
* A hot water bottle in a towel held against the swollen glands can ease the pain.

GP:
Contact your GP to confirm diagnosis.

There is no cure for mumps. Your doctor may advise paracetamol for any pain that is present, be it in the swollen glands, tummy or testes. Call your GP if there is any headache with neck stiffness, or if you are worried.

FEVER CONTROL

Too many parents do the WRONG thing when their child has a raised temperature. They keep the child warm with lots of blankets on the bed. The windows are kept closed and the heating is on because it is thought that the child should sweat the fever out of the system!

This is totally WRONG, and is in fact VERY DANGEROUS!

The child with a fever has a raised temperature and should, therefore, be COOLED DOWN, because a raised temperature can cause the child's brain to overheat, and when this happens the child could have a convulsion or fit!

This is a frightening sight for any parent and can easily be prevented by correctly controlling the fever, so that the child's temperature is brought down, NOT sent even higher. This type of fit is called a 'febrile convulsion'.

Here is a simple easy-to-remember fever control guide.

* COOL ROOM
  – open a window, turn the heating OFF. If possible put an electric fan in the room.

* COOL SPONGE
– sponge your child's head, neck and arms with a sponge or cloth soaked in cool water. If the child is prone to febrile convulsions, cool-sponging the whole body will be necessary to get the temperature right down.

* COOL DRINKS
– plenty of cool or iced drinks. Whatever your child fancies, but avoid 'fizzy' drinks as these may cause vomiting if the child is feeling nauseated.

* COOL BEDDING
– probably one sheet with maybe a light blanket is all that is necessary. The child may even kick those off if he is uncomfortable. No duvets and no electric blankets!

* PARACETAMOL SYRUP
– NOT aspirin. It has been found that a rare serious condition called Reye's syndrome seems to be more common in children taking aspirin. Therefore, NEVER give aspirin or medicines containing aspirin to any child under the age of 12 years. Use paracetamol syrup, following the dosage instructions on the bottle for your child's age group.

* ANTIBIOTICS
– if your child has been given antibiotics by the doctor do ensure that the full course is taken, even if the child is appearing better within a couple of days. Most antibiotics should be taken for a period of 5 days.

SO DON'T FORGET:
Cool room – cool sponge – cool drinks – cool bedding PLUS paracetamol syrup and, maybe, antibiotics.

EARS, NOSE & THROAT

EARS

The commonest ear infections are:
* Otitis (*oh-tite-iss*) externa
* Otitis media (*mee-dee-ya*)
* Serous (*see-russ*) otitis media

OTITIS EXTERNA

What is otitis externa?
Otitis externa is inflammation of the outer part of the ear. The skin is often flaky, reddened and the inflammation extends down into

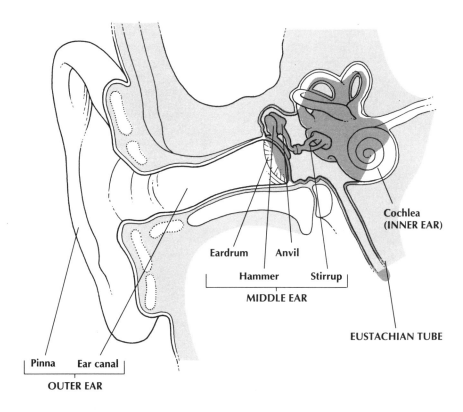

Eardrum   Anvil

Hammer   Stirrup

MIDDLE EAR

Cochlea
(INNER EAR)

EUSTACHIAN TUBE

Pinna   Ear canal

OUTER EAR

the ear canal. If the skin becomes infected the ear can become moist with discharge, cracked and very tender.

Who gets otitis externa?
It occurs more commonly in children with eczema, psoriasis, seborrhoeic dermatitis or other widespread skin disorder.

What causes otitis externa?
It is caused by infection of the skin with bacteria, viruses or fungi.

Can you prevent otitis externa?
There are no specific measures. In children who are to have their ears pierced at a very early stage it is recommended that the earrings be made only of pure gold, as a reaction to the metal, nickel, which is often present in cheaper jewellery, can cause a reaction that results in otitis externa.

Any severe reaction around the holes in the pierced ear lobes may necessitate a course of oral antibiotics.

How should you treat otitis externa?
Your GP will prescribe the necessary treatment in the form of ear drops, usually containing an antibiotic or antifungal agent to kill off the offending organism. If the

HOW TO INSERT EAR DROPS

First of all warm the drops, gently, in the hands.

Allow 3 or 4 drops to enter the canal into the ear, whilst the child rests his head to one side.

Gentle massage of the tragus, the area directly in front of the ear opening, will cause the drops to reach much deeper into the ear canal (see diagram). Often the drops will contain a mild steroid to bring the inflammation of the skin under control.

infection only involves the pinna of the ear (the ear lobe) an ointment or cream will be prescribed.

OTITIS MEDIA

What is otitis media?
Otitis media is an infection of the middle ear, see diagram opposite.

Symptoms

* The child is obviously unwell.
* The child is feverish.
* The child is in pain. The pain of otitis media can be severe and the child will scream out, often holding the affected ear. In younger children they often pull or rub the ear in the early stages of the disease. Thereafter, even touching the ear can cause severe pain.
* Pus and/or blood may be seen in the ear, or on the child's pillow.
* The child may be deaf on the affected side. If treatment is soon started, this is not usually a permanent deafness. The hearing returns once the infection has cleared up.

Who gets otitis media?
Otitis media often comes on during a cold-like illness, measles or throat infections.

What causes otitis media?
Otitis media is caused by a bacterial or viral infection getting into the middle ear cavity, often from the throat or nose. Younger children up to the age of 4 are more prone to otitis media, because infections in the throat and nasal passages easily spread along the eustachian tube, which is much shorter in younger children. The diagram on page 52 shows how the eustachian tube connects the nasal passages with the cavity of the middle ear.

Can you prevent otitis media?
It has been thought that bottle feeding a baby in the recumbent position (lying flat), causes the baby to be more prone to milk being aspirated up the baby's short eustachian tube, with resultant irritation of the middle ear – so sit your baby up when bottle feeding him!

Otitis media is more common in homes where babies and children are exposed to cigarette smoke.

REMEMBER

Any child with earache should have his ears examined.

Children are fond of putting all sorts of little items into their ears!

54

It is very important that the condition is treated promptly, to prevent complications occurring. Complications can include long term deafness and, before the days of antibiotics, spread of the infection from the ears to the brain, which is only half an inch away, was a serious consequence, resulting in brain abscess and meningitis.

How should you treat otitis media?
Yourself:
CONTACT YOUR GP

Do not go poking anything into the ear, and do not put any eardrops into the affected ear.

Your child may get relief from resting the ear on a warm hot-water bottle covered with a soft blanket.

Paracetamol syrup will help to relieve the pain.

GP:
Your GP will examine the ear to find the cause of the problem – not an easy thing to do when the poor child is screaming with pain and defending his sore ear from invasion by a total stranger, apparently intent on causing even more suffering by pulling on the throbbing ear and sticking a torch right inside it!

An antibiotic medicine will often be prescribed, to be taken on a regular basis along with pain-relieving paracetamol syrup. The preferred antibiotic for this condition is amoxycillin, or if the child is allergic to penicillin, co-trimoxazole, erythromycin or cefaclor are used.

Decongestants are of no use in this condition.

CAUSES OF EARACHE

Infection of the outer ear – otitis externa.
Infection of the middle ear – otitis media.
Boil in the ear.
Foreign bodies in the ear – e.g. little beads.
Injury or bang on the ear.
Throat infection/tonsillitis.
Mumps.
Toothache.

SEROUS OTITIS MEDIA

What is serous otitis media?
This condition is also known as glue ear. Glue ear can cause deafness. Deafness often goes unnoticed by parents and schoolteachers, yet even slight loss of hearing can have devastating

55

effects upon a child's development, speech, language and learning ability. I feel very strongly that not enough emphasis is given to the severe problems that this condition produces.

With glue ear, the middle ear is filled with a fluid that can be thin or thick in consistency. Often there are no symptoms whatsoever – no earache, or discharge from the ear. Older children may complain of deafness, a pressure in the ear or a ringing or popping in the ears.

Who gets serous otitis media?

This condition usually occurs in children under the age of 12 years.

It appears more common in children who have:
* Recurring middle ear infections.
* Recurring colds and nasal infections.
* Recurring coughs and chest infections.
* Allergies, e.g. hay fever.
* Eustachian tube problems.
* Parents who smoke.
* Cleft palate.
* Down's syndrome.

PARTIAL DEAFNESS IN CHILDREN IS EXTREMELY COMMON

What causes serous otitis media?

The exact cause is not clear. It appears that those children who develop this condition have been unable to equalise the pressure between their middle ear and the atmosphere, due to blockage in their eustachian tubes. The decrease in pressure in the middle ear results in an outpouring of fluid. This hinders the conduction of sound across the middle ear into the inner ear, where sound signals would normally be received and transmitted to the brain.

However, in many cases glue ear tends to clear up itself, in time, as the child grows.

ALL CHILDREN WITH THE FOLLOWING PROBLEMS SHOULD HAVE THEIR HEARING TESTED:

Speech difficulties.
Poor progress in school.
Problems with behaviour.
Recurring earache.
Cleft palate.

How can you prevent serous otitis media?

* By paying prompt attention to the treatment of those recurring infections listed above.
* By not exposing your baby or child to cigarette smoke in the home.

How should you treat serous otitis media?
Yourself:
If you think your child is not hearing too well, try the 'whisper test'. When behind him quietly call his name, first on one side then on the other. If there is no response there may well be a hearing problem that needs further assessment – consult your GP.

GP:
Your GP will examine your child's ear drum with a special torch. If there is evidence of glue ear, the child is best referred to an ENT (ear, nose and throat) specialist, for full hearing assessment and examination.

ENT specialist:
He may decide to admit your child to hospital to drain off the fluid from the middle ear, and to insert a 'grommet' into the ear drum. A grommet is basically a tiny drainage tube, made of plastic, which allows fluid inside the ear to drain out. This prevents any further blockage within the ear and hearing is restored. The grommets often fall out after 6–9 months when the ears have returned to normal. Most children or parents are never aware that the grommets have come out, as they are so small. If they do not fall out the ENT doctor will remove them when he sees your child at his routine follow-up appointment in the out-patient clinic. Your child CAN go swimming with grommets in the ear. If you want to be ultra-cautious, then a bathing cap or good ear plugs will be effective in stopping water causing any problems.

Hence, the basic treatment of glue ear is directed at restoring the child's hearing to normal. As the child grows the condition clears due to lengthening of the eustachian tube.

NOSE

NOSEBLEEDS

What are nosebleeds?
The medical term for a nosebleed is an epistaxis. Most nosebleeds arise from blood vessels at the front of the nasal septum, the piece of

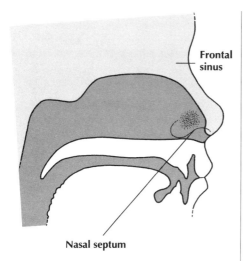

Frontal
sinus

Nasal septum

cartilage that separates the nostrils (see diagram).

Who gets nosebleeds?

Nosebleeds can occur at any age, but are common in children and often no obvious cause for them can be found. They frequently occur at night and the poor child wakes up with his pillow and face covered in what appears to be vast quantities of blood. It always looks worse than it really is.

What causes nosebleeds?

* Picking the nose.
* A bang to the nose.
* A foreign body up the nose.
* A bout of coughing or sneezing.
* The common cold, sinusitis or hay fever.

* Blood disorders, where blood clotting ability is affected.
* No obvious reason.

How can you prevent nosebleeds?

Try to dissuade nose picking – it is about all you can do!

How should you treat nosebleeds?

Yourself:
Sit your child down with their head bent FORWARD over a bowl or a sink. Tilting the head back causes blood to go down the back of the nose into the throat where it may be swallowed into the stomach. This can result in making the child feel sick and actually vomit.

Do NOT pack the nose with tissue or cotton wool! Do not put anything into the nose. It may help initially to stop the bleeding, but when the packing is removed bleeding may start again as the clots are disrupted.

Tell the child to breathe through his open mouth.

Firmly pinch the soft flesh just above the nostrils – NOT the bridge of the nose. Compression of this lower part of the nose causes direct pressure on the blood vessels that are leaking. This stops the bleeding and helps clot formation within the leaking vessels. The nostrils must

58

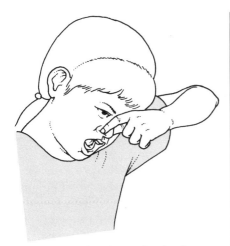

be pinched for about 5–10 minutes – without letting go! It may not be a long time but it seems like an eternity – especially to the child who has to sit still and breathe only through his mouth. A useful hint here is to get the child to hold a cork between their teeth. This keeps the mouth open and gives them something to concentrate on whilst waiting for the bleeding to stop! After 5–10 minutes, slowly remove your fingers from the child's nose and make sure that they do not rub the nose, blow it, or pick it, as such actions might cause further bleeding. Be gentle with that nose! If bleeding is not controlled by these measures – contact your GP.

GP:
Your GP may attempt the same procedure of digital nasal compression. In the rare instances that this fails your child may have to be seen by an ENT specialist at your local hospital. After an inspection of the nose the ENT doctor may use a special nasal dressing that will probably control the bleeding. If the bleeding is caused by a prominent and fragile blood vessel, then that may be cauterised under a general anaesthetic. Cauterisation involves touching the affected vessel with a special type of heat probe which immediately seals the leak and coagulates the blood.

THROAT

TONSILLITIS

What is tonsillitis?
Tonsillitis is an infection of the tonsils which are situated at the back of the mouth, one on each side of the throat.

The tonsils are really guards or custodians at the oral entrance to the body. They are unable to filter out airborne organisms but they are exposed to germs and invading bacteria in the air, food and drink as they pass through the mouth. Contact with invading and infecting organisms causes the tonsils to enlarge and stimulate the body's defence mechanism – the immune system – to produce antibodies to attack the invading germs. As the tonsils become infected, so the glands in the neck and under the lower jaw react, becoming tender and enlarged. All this is part of the body's defence system coming into action when faced with threatening germs, such as bacteria and viruses.

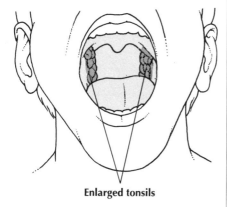

Enlarged tonsils

The symptoms

* A very sore throat.
* A fever.
* Difficulty in swallowing and feeling very ill.
* Loss of appetite.
* Enlarged reddened tonsils with spots of yellow or white pus.
* Enlarged glands in the neck, just under the angle of the jaw. These glands are tender and can cause restriction of neck movements.

* Bad breath.
* Sometimes abdominal (tummy) pain. This occurs as a result of infecting organisms being swallowed in the saliva. As the glands swell in the neck, so do glands inside the abdomen as they try to combat the infecting organisms inside the intestines. Swelling of abdominal glands is known as mesenteric adenitis (see page 66). Diarrhoea can also result from the germs entering the intestines or bowels.

Who gets tonsillitis?
Tonsillitis is rare in children under 1 year old, and not so common in those children over 10 years. It is at its most common in children aged 4–12 years of age – the school years. At school they often meet infections for the first time, and this exposure to more and more infectious organisms helps to develop their resistance, so attacks of tonsillitis become less common as the child gets older.

What are adenoids?
The adenoids lie right at the back of the nose, above the level of the palate, so they cannot be seen.

The adenoids are made up of the

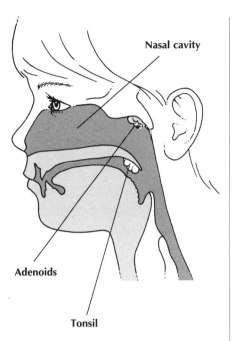

Nasal cavity

Adenoids

Tonsil

What causes tonsillitis?

The commonest cause of true tonsillitis is a bacterium known as haemolytic streptococcus. This bacterium is the cause of two very unusual complications – nephritis and rheumatic fever. But don't be too concerned as these are rare conditions.

Viruses can also cause tonsillitis, but in such circumstances there is rarely any pus to be seen on the surface of the enlarged tonsils.

Can you prevent tonsillitis?

It is very difficult to do. It is almost part of the growing up process.

How should you treat tonsillitis?
Yourself:

* Check if there is a fever.
* Look in your child's throat. The tonsils can be seen easier if you get your child to say 'aah', whilst you gently press on the tongue with a spoon handle. If the tonsils look red, enlarged or are covered with yellow spots contact your GP.

same kind of tissue as the tonsils and they serve the same function – to protect the body against infecting organisms, especially those that enter through the nose. Tonsils become enlarged and so do the adenoids. Enlarged adenoids can block the back of the nasal passages, so that the child is unable to breathe through the nose. This produces snoring and mouth-breathing. Big adenoids can also block the eustachian tube that connects the ear with the nasal cavity. Such a problem often leads to recurring ear infections and glue ear (see page 55).

GP:

On confirming the diagnosis, your GP will probably prescribe a course of antibiotics. The antibiotics most commonly-used are penicillin, amoxycillin, erythromycin and cefaclor. Paracetamol syrup will help to lower the temperature and ease the pain and soreness.

Tonsillectomy

This is the commonest operation performed on children. 75% of all tonsillectomies are performed in the under 16s.

Sometimes the tonsils are removed with the adenoids – medically known as a 'T and A' (tonsillectomy and adenoidectomy). There is, however, less tendency to rush into removing tonsils these days.

Strong reasons for removing the tonsils are:

* Extreme enlargement causing blockage to the child's airways.
* Recurring tonsillitis, causing febrile convulsions (fever fits or fits due to high temperature).
* Recurring tonsillitis of great frequency – more than 4 attacks in the past 12 months.

Your child will probably be admitted into hospital the night before the operation and, all being well, will be discharged the day after surgery. As the throat is very sore after this operation, fluids, soups, liquidised and soft foods are recommended for the first couple of days. A period of two weeks of convalescence is advisable.

Remember that all operations carry a certain degree of risk, and do respect your ENT specialist's opinion if he is against removing your child's tonsils.

TUMMY TROUBLES

Tummy pain or abdominal pain, as your doctor may call it, can be caused by many different conditions. Here is a list of the more common ones that are encountered:

* Appendicitis
* Mesenteric Adenitis (*mee-zent-erik adden-eye-tis*)
* Colic
* Gastroenteritis

APPENDICITIS

What is appendicitis?
Appendicitis is the inflammation of the appendix. The appendix is a narrow little tube lying on the right side of the abdomen, just above the groin region.

The human body has two areas of intestine, the small intestine and the large intestine (see diagram).

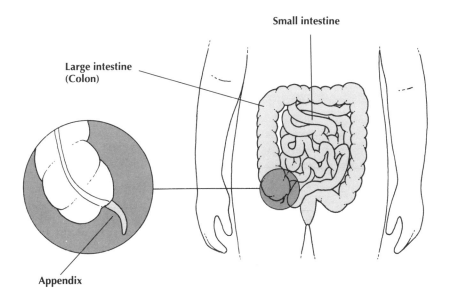

Small intestine

Large intestine (Colon)

Appendix

The appendix is attached to the large intestine close to the junction of the small and large intestines.

The appendix seems to serve no purpose whatsoever in humans. It is shaped like a worm with only one open end at it's junction with the large intestine. Because it is a dead-end it can easily become blocked and inflamed. This inflammation causes swelling and infection of the appendix. When this happens, pain is felt and the patient can become quite ill.

The symptoms of appendicitis are as follows:

* Tummy pain. The pain often starts near to the navel (umbilicus or 'belly button'). The pain comes and goes. After a few hours the pain settles into the lower right-hand corner of the abdomen. By this time the pain has become more of a severe constant ache. Touching the abdomen makes the pain worse and any movement, such as sitting up or turning, is extremely painful. The pain can be so severe that the child lies very still.

* The child feels sick and often does vomit.

* The child is feverish and flushed.

* The tongue is coated and the breath may smell.

* The child is usually off his food and may refuse drinks.

* Sometimes there can be diarrhoea or constipation.

Who gets appendicitis?
Appendicitis is rare in infants under 1 year of age. It is the commonest surgical emergency, though having said that only about 200 people per 100,000 (1 per 500) are affected each year.

What causes appendicitis?
As mentioned above, blockage of the narrow open end of the appendix causes it to become inflamed. Bacteria trapped inside the appendix multiply and infection causes pus to build up inside it. If the appendix swells further it bursts and the infecting bacteria spread into the abdominal cavity to cause peritonitis – a serious emergency. It is thought that blockage of the appendix is produced more commonly by a lump of hard faeces. In rare

circumstances a clump of worms such as threadworms have been found to be obstructing the opening of the appendix.

Can you prevent appendicitis?
There is no way we can prevent appendicitis. Obviously avoiding constipation and getting prompt treatment for threadworms (see page 126) may help.

How should you treat appendicitis?
Yourself:
You cannot treat appendicitis in the home. If your child has tummy pains for more than 2 hours contact your doctor. If your child has tummy pains with a temperature you MUST get in touch with your doctor. In fact, if your child has any sort of tummy pain which is causing him some distress always call your GP for advice.

Once you contact your doctor, don't give your child anything by mouth in case he has to have a general anaesthetic for the removal of his appendix.

GP:
If your GP diagnoses appendicitis, your child will be admitted to hospital, where once the diagnosis is confirmed the appendix will be removed. The operation is called an appendicectomy (*a-pen-diss-ekt-ummy*).

If your little one is to be admitted into hospital for an appendicectomy ask at the hospital if you can stay with your child. More and more hospitals are providing this type of facility as it is very reassuring for the child to have Mum (or Dad) with them during their stay in their strange new surroundings.

The operation is a straightforward procedure, and even if they find that the appendix is not inflamed at the time of the operation the surgeon will still remove it so that your child will not have to face possible appendicitis in the future. This is done because the appendix has no function in the body, so when it is removed we do not miss it!

Within 24 hours of the operation the child is allowed light food and drinks. After 3–4 days most children are allowed home, and then the stitches (sutures) are removed 7–10 days after the operation. Taking the stitches out is not usually a painful procedure, in fact it can often make the child feel a lot more comfortable, because stitches themselves can pull tightly on the skin and can dig into the skin. The hospital will ask you to take your child either to the outpatient department or to your GP for removal of the stitches. If there are no complications your child will be able to resume full normal activities about 4 weeks after the operation.

MESENTERIC ADENITIS

What is mesenteric adenitis?

This condition, sometimes known as mesenteric lymphadenitis, is a condition where glands inside the abdomen become inflamed and swollen, causing pains in the abdomen. The glandular swelling is quite similar to the enlargement of the neck glands that occurs when a throat infection is present.

The glands, which are known as lymph glands, become swollen as a result of blocking the attack of invading organisms which have entered the body in the throat area or, in the case of mesenteric adenitis, through the intestine. A child with an infected throat or cough or cold cannot avoid swallowing infecting organisms from the throat area. Once these 'bugs' are in the intestines they try to invade the body by passing through the wall of the intestines but find their progress blocked by the body's defence mechanisms – the lymph glands. In response to this attack the glands swell up and can become inflamed, causing pain in the abdomen.

The pain can be very similar to the pain of appendicitis. It is often in the centre of the abdomen. There may also be a slight fever. However, the child is not as ill as the child with appendicitis.

Who gets mesenteric adenitis?

Any child. Though it is more common in children who have a throat infection, cough, cold, sinusitis, chest infection or even ear infection.

Can you prevent mesenteric adenitis?

No, the condition cannot be prevented.

How should you treat mesenteric adenitis?
Yourself:
DON'T try to make the diagnosis yourself. Always get your GP to see your child when there is any doubt about what is causing tummy pain. Once the doctor has confirmed that it is nothing more serious he will probably treat the pre-existing condition. If your child has a throat or chest infection you will probably receive an antibiotic.

Differences between APPENDICITIS and MESENTERIC ADENITIS.

APPENDICITIS	MESENTERIC ADENITIS
Pain	
Starts around the navel.	Often starts around the navel and may stay in that location.
Settles in right hand corner of abdomen (patient's right side).	More often stays in central part of abdomen. May settle in right hand corner of abdomen.
May be so severe that child is unable to move or turn.	Rarely that severe.
Abdomen is tender to touch. Pressing on abdomen causes pain to worsen.	Abdomen rarely tender to touch.
Temperature	
Child nearly always has a marked fever, and is flushed.	Only mild fever, if any. Rarely flushed.
Degree of Illness	
Child is obviously ill. Is off food and often vomiting.	Child may have another infection such as a sore throat, cough or cold. He rarely vomits or is off his food.

Simple pain relief in the form of paracetamol will also be recommended until the condition has cleared. If there is a fever see the recommendations on fever control on page 50, remembering to give your child plenty of fluids.

GP:
As mesenteric adenitis commonly mimics appendicitis, it can sometimes be a difficult condition to diagnose. Your GP may be concerned about the exact cause of your child's tummy pain and may

send your child down to the paediatrician (specialist in children's diseases) at your local hospital. Keeping the child in hospital for observation and simple blood tests will help to ensure the correct diagnosis. It sometimes happens that the child is diagnosed as having appendicitis and is taken to theatre for an appendicectomy only for the appendix to be found to be normal whilst the glands are found to be enlarged! The surgeon will remove the appendix but the mesenteric glands are left alone.

COLIC

What is colic?

The colic that affects babies is a condition where there appears to be an episode of abdominal pain, occurring more often in the evening between 5 pm and 10 pm. During the day the baby is usually not in pain, feeds well, sleeps well and is otherwise a fit healthy baby. During the attack the baby appears to be in intense pain, crying or screaming, as he draws his legs up to his tummy. His face is often red and he is obviously very upset!

The pain can last up to 2 or 3 hours and then wears off. The condition is harmless to the baby as it clears up by the time the baby is 4 months old, but it is very disturbing for the parents during that period of time.

Who gets colic?

* Colic is common in babies up to the age of 3–4 months, it is often referred to as 'three-month colic'. It is not a condition of older children.
* It is more common in bottle-fed babies.
* It is more common in babies who are given cow's milk.
* It is more common in babies who are given solids very early.
* It is more common in the babies of smoking mothers.

What causes colic?

Despite colic being a common condition affecting so many young babies, we still do not know the real cause of this complaint. It is thought to be a spasm of the baby's intestines, maybe due to an irregularity in the intestines which have not yet learned how to function correctly.

During the baby's development in the womb, there was no feeding through the mouth and there was, therefore, no great activity in the baby's bowels or intestines.

After birth the baby starts taking in nourishing feeds every few hours, and it is thought that along with the feed, the baby swallows substantial amounts of air into the stomach and intestines. The bowel tries to cope with this new experience as best it can, but does not 'get its act together', and is not able to coordinate correctly its complex actions of gently moving on the contents of the intestines in a smooth and regular fashion. So air and gas get trapped in parts of the bowel and the intestines contract down in a haphazard and often painful manner in an attempt to move the contents on in the best way possible. As the intestines mature and learn to act smoothly (and painlessly) through their daily contact with air and food, so the condition gradually settles.

Can you prevent colic?

* Whether you baby is breast-fed or bottle-fed, always stop half way through a feed and burp him by patting gently on his back, or rubbing his back as you sit him upright with him facing over your shoulder. A hungry baby will greedily feed on breast or bottle and often swallow a lot of air, along with the milk. That swallowed air may cause him some colicky discomfort later. If your baby does not bring up any wind within a couple of minutes put him back to feed, otherwise he may start crying, get upset and swallow air, thus producing more colic!

* Try to breast feed your baby at least for the first 3 months, if you can.

* If you are bottle feeding, make sure that the hole in the teat is the right size. Hold the bottle upside down, and if the milk drops at a slow steady rate from the teat – that's about right! If no drops drip out, the hole is too small and if the milk runs out, the teat hole is too large. Always ensure that you are holding the bottle at the correct angle, i.e. so that the teat is always full of milk and the baby is not sucking air from above the milk.

* Do not offer your baby any solid food until he is 3 months old. The baby's immature intestines may find it difficult to cope with

69

the new proteins and substances presented by some solid or semi-solid foodstuffs until he is older than 3 months.

* Do NOT give your baby ordinary cow's milk until he is 12 months old.

* When you are weaning him you may find that certain baby foods disagree with him and may cause colic. In that situation avoid the offending foods – there are plenty more to choose from.

THE DANISH 'TUMMY RUB'

A team of Danish doctors has found that gently massaging the baby's tummy after a feed has brought about a great deal of relief with colicky babies.

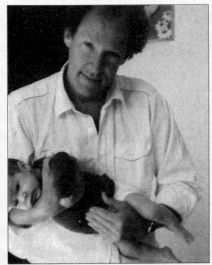

Holding the baby as shown, softly massage his tummy with the ends of the fingers of the left hand, using not the tips of the fingers but the pulp or fleshy parts of the fingers.

Massage in a circular, clockwise direction, starting in small circles close to the navel and gradually making larger circles with firmer pressure.

Doing this for about 10 minutes after each feed stimulates the intestine and the baby passes

Photograph courtesy of Dr Jan-Helge Larsen wind and also moves his bowels.

Try this simple procedure, it can be remarkably effective.

How should you treat colic?
Yourself:
* Wind or burp him to see if that will help.

* Try to soothe your baby by:
  – rocking him
  – cuddling him
  – walking to and fro, whilst cuddling
  – walking him in the pram
  – singing to him
  – playing gentle music to him
  – bathing him
  – putting the carrycot in the car and taking him for a drive.

* Gripe water sometimes helps, but to be honest, there is no scientific evidence that this has any effect upon infant colic.

GP:
Once your doctor has made sure that nothing more serious is happening there is little he can do from the medical point of view.

The only preparation that I know of that is officially indicated for use in the treatment of infant colic in babies under 6 months is a liquid called *Infacol*. Give between 0.5ml to 1ml just before each feed. This can be bought over the counter and is also available on prescription. It can safely be used in babies under 6 months.

A baby older than 6 months that is having bouts of colic may be helped with a preparation called *Merbentyl* syrup, which is given 15 minutes before feeds. This is available only on prescription and your own GP will advise on its suitability for your baby. It must not be given to babies under 6 months.

If you are exhausted by your baby's screaming fits, DO contact your doctor, and explain that you are at the end of your tether. You must explain how totally drained you have become, for you may need further help or support to get you through this difficult time.

GASTROENTERITIS, DIARRHOEA AND VOMITING

What is gastroenteritis?
Gastroenteritis is inflammation of the stomach (gastritis) and of the intestines (enteritis). The inflammation of the stomach causes vomiting and the inflammation of the intestines or bowels causes the 'runs' or diarrhoea. The diarrhoea can be profuse, loose, watery stools, smelling absolutely foul and can be

71

any colour from light brown to yellow or green. The younger the child the more serious is this condition, therefore this section concentrates on gastroenteritis in the little baby.

Symptoms

* Diarrhoea
* Vomiting
* Nausea
* Fever
* Tummy pains
* Not feeding

Gastroenteritis is a very important condition in babies, because it can rapidly become very serious, leading to dehydration. The baby is unable to retain his feeds because of the vomiting, and in vomiting he is also losing fluid from his own stomach. The diarrhoea obviously results in loss of further fluid from the baby's intestines, and because babies are so small, their bodies have very little storage capacity for extra fluids. In the fluids that are lost, the baby is also losing important substances that are needed for vital functions in the body, these substances are known as electrolytes and minerals.

Once dehydration sets in it can become a life-threatening situation.

SIGNS OF DEHYDRATION IN A BABY

* The baby's lips, tongue and mouth are dry.
* The baby's urine is dark yellow.
* The baby is passing little urine.
* The fontanelle is sunken (see diagram).
* The baby is weak and floppy.
* The baby shows few signs of interest in his surroundings.
* The baby's eyes may look more prominent.
* The baby's skin becomes more lax and less elastic.

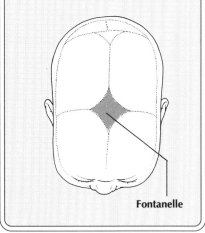

Fontanelle

72

• DEHYDRATION SIGNS
  IN A BABY ARE
  DANGEROUS.

• THIS IS AN EMERGENCY
  SITUATION.
  CONTACT YOUR
  DOCTOR AT ONCE.

• IF HE IS NOT AVAILABLE
  GET YOUR BABY
  TO HOSPITAL
  IMMEDIATELY.

Who gets gastroenteritis?
Anyone – baby, toddler, child or adult. None of us are immune. However, it certainly is more common in babies who are bottle-fed. Any baby in a household where there is already a case of gastroenteritis will also be at higher risk of catching the disease.

What causes gastroenteritis?
Gastroenteritis is usually the result of an infection by either a virus, a bacterium or a parasite.

In babies the commonest cause of this condition is a virus infection. The virus can be transmitted in the air, it does not have to be passed on by direct personal contact. So if the virus is in the air it could just settle and multiply on a baby's dirty bottle, or in the baby's milk if it is not freshly prepared.

The gastroenteritis caused by bacteria is more common in adults and is known as food-poisoning. In this situation the bacteria get into the body directly from eating food which contains the offending bacteria. These bugs usually get into the food from an infected person not adequately washing their hands after going to the toilet.

Gastroenteritis caused by a parasite is known as dysentery, but this is rare in this country.

Can you prevent gastroenteritis?

* Breast feed your baby if you can. Your breast milk cannot become contaminated with viruses from the atmosphere like bottle milk can. Your breast milk also gives the baby resistance to all sorts of infections by passing on maternal antibodies to the baby.

* If you are bottle feeding you MUST pay meticulous attention to sterilisation procedures when cleaning the baby's feeding containers and when preparing the baby's feeds.

Read the section of this book on feeding (page 10) to see the importance of feed preparation. What is convenient for you (for example in preparing several feeds at once) may prove very dangerous for your baby.
* Discard all unfinished feeds.
* Do not leave bottles or teats lying around in the open air between feeds. Put them in the sterilising tank with sterilising fluid.
* Ensure that everyone in the house always washes their hands after being on the toilet – whether there is gastroenteritis in the house or not!
* Anyone with gastroenteritis should be treated promptly and should have as little contact with babies or little ones as possible.
* Anyone with gastroenteritis should keep their own towels to themselves.

How should you treat gastroenteritis?
The most important aspect of treating this condition is to maintain fluid and electrolyte intake in the child, to prevent dehydration. Although you can do this yourself,

following the advice given below, I have to emphasise that you MUST contact your doctor in any of the following situations:

* If you are worried AT ALL about your baby with vomiting and/or diarrhoea.
* If your baby has had vomiting AND diarrhoea for 4 hours, before electrolyte replacement has even commenced.
* If your baby is not improving after 4–6 hours of any electrolyte replacement that you have started yourself.
* If your baby has diarrhoea only and has not responded to 24 hours of electrolyte replacement fluid.
* If your baby develops signs of dehydration at ANY time (see page 72).

Yourself:
Once your baby starts with vomiting and/or diarrhoea, stop bottle feeding him with his usual feed and immediately switch him to what's called an electrolyte replacement solution. There are, at present, three brands of these solutions on the market:
Dioralyte
Electrolade
Rehidrat

GASTROENTERITIS AND BABIES

THE YOUNGER THE BABY, THE MORE DANGEROUS THIS CONDITION IS.

(And the older the child the less dangerous. Look how often we, as adults, have the runs without any serious problems!)

THE MORE RUNNY THE DIARRHOEA, THE MORE FLUID IS LOST.

IF YOUR BABY IS VOMITING AND HAS DIARRHOEA, HE IS LOSING FLUID FROM BOTH ENDS, AND IS NOT GETTING NOURISHMENT INTO HIS BODY.

These solutions are all excellent methods of replacing lost fluids and excellent sources of the necessary electrolytes your baby will need. They come as powders which have to be mixed with water that has been boiled and allowed to cool. They come in assorted flavours, including citrus, blackcurrant, banana, melon, lemon/lime, orange, and plain. All can be bought over the counter at your chemist's shop, and they are also available on prescription.

The following instructions should be followed:

* Make up a solution of the powder as directed on the sachet.
* Completely replace your baby's feeds with an equivalent volume of the made-up electrolyte solution. So if you baby was to have had 5oz of milk feed, give him 5oz of the fluid replacement. Do NOT give him any of his normal feed. He may well feel hungry and may cry because he is hungry, but his stomach and intestines must be given a chance to rest and recover from this infection.
* If your baby is being breast-fed, give him a 5–6oz electrolyte drink in a bottle immediately after a breast feed. If he is vomiting and not keeping down his breast feed, then stop breast feeding and give him only electrolyte replacement feeds – as

75

much as he'll take at each feed.

* In cases of diarrhoea AND vomiting continue with this routine for about 4-6 hours – if there is no sign of improvement call the doctor.
* In cases of diarrhoea ONLY, continue with this routine for up to 24 hours. If there is no improvement call the doctor.
* You can make up your own electrolyte replacement fluid quite simply at home. The ingredients should be:
  – 4 teaspoons of glucose (or sugar)
  – 1 teaspoon of salt
  – 1 pint of water (boiled)

REMEMBER: IF YOU ARE WORRIED TALK TO YOUR DOCTOR FOR HELP AND ADVICE.

GP:

Your doctor will probably advise you on the use of the oral electrolyte replacement fluids which have been described above. As the child improves he will advise you to gradually re-introduce your child to its previous feeds in a gradual routine, probably by giving the baby quarter-strength feeds, for a couple of feeds, followed by half-strength feeds, then three-quarter-strength feeds and finally right back to normal.

Sometimes with older children your doctor may prescribe an anti-diarrhoea medicine and even an anti-vomiting medicine, though these are not usually the first-choice treatments as most children respond to the electrolyte fluids which are safe, simple and have no side effects.

If your doctor feels that your child has not responded quickly enough to treatment, he may recommend that the baby is admitted to hospital. Don't worry too much about this situation as we doctors tend to be ultra-cautious when it comes to little babies with gastroenteritis. Better to err on the side of caution.

In hospital the doctors will ensure that your baby is given full fluid replacement by using an intravenous drip to pour fluid directly into the body. Small sips of fluid may also be given by mouth and your child will soon be improving. You will most likely be allowed to stay with your baby in hospital.

76

BED-WETTING

What is bed-wetting?

The medical term for bed-wetting is nocturnal enuresis, which is defined as the involuntary passage of urine (enuresis) at night (nocturnal) in a child over the age of 5 years, in the absence of any physical cause in the urinary system or nervous system. So you'll see that we only consider treating it as a problem when the child is still bed-wetting over the age of 5 years.

No treatment will normally be offered in an under 5 year-old. Sometimes a child may have been dry for many months and starts to wet the bed again, this is called secondary enuresis.

Daytime control of the bladder is usually gained at 1–4 years.

Night-time control is normally gained at 2–5 years.

75% of children will be dry at night, by the age of 4 years, and 80–85% before they are 5 years old.

> Between 15% and 20% of normal 5 year olds will wet the bed at least twice a week.
>
> Only 2% of 12 year olds wet the bed.

Who gets the condition?

More than 500,000 children between the ages of 6 and 16 have a bed-wetting problem. So do not feel that your child is alone and abnormal, bed-wetting is quite an ordinary problem which is nothing for you or your child to be ashamed of. The good news is that it will clear up; most children respond to treatment for this condition. Over 70,000 adults between 20 and 25 also have this problem. There is a strong connection between your child having the problem, and someone in the family also suffering or having suffered from enuresis. Members of the same family often stop bed-wetting at about the same age. However, the fact that the child will spontaneously be clear of the problem in time is not very helpful to the mother who is burdened with the daily and relentless toil of dealing with sodden sheets, blankets and mattresses. Nor is this reassurance impressive to little Johnny who wants to go camping with the cubs, but can't because of his problem! Well the good news is "There's no need to suffer" as there are some very effective treatments available for this problem – see *Can you prevent bed-wetting?* opposite.

BED-WETTING 'FILE O' FACTS'

Bed-wetting occurs more commonly in:

* Boys.
* First-born children.
* Families where there is someone with a bed-wetting problem.
* Children with learning difficulties.
* Children with delayed development.
* Children in socially-deprived families.

What causes bed-wetting?

There seems to be no specific abnormality in the bladder, kidneys or the nerves that supply these organs in most children who have a bed-wetting problem. They may be genetically predisposed to getting the problem, because of a family history of enuresis, but intense investigation will show no abnormalities whatsoever in most cases.

However, all children with this problem should have their GP or bladder specialist eliminate certain conditions such as:

* Infection of the kidneys or bladder.
* Constipation.
* Congenital abnormalities of the urinary tract (waterworks).
* Diabetes.
* Stress at home or school.

In rare circumstances the bed-wetting will be due to one of these causes, but in most cases a child who bedwets is normal both physically and mentally.

Can you prevent bed-wetting?

There are 4 methods of treating bed-wetting: General Advice, Reward System, Alarm Method, Medicines.

General Advice

NEVER scold a child for a wet night. The child cannot help it, he is asleep when he empties his bladder. Disciplining could make the child anxious and hence make the problem worse.

Praise him for every night he is dry, and say nothing about the wet nights.

Explain to him that he is not alone with this little problem (half a million other children are bed-wetting each night) and that he is not abnormal in any way.

Restricting VOLUME of fluids is NOT necessary.

Restricting TYPES of fluids IS necessary. Certain drinks contain substances known as xanthines, such as caffeine, which are diuretics, that is, they make us pass water. So during the evening DON'T give your child tea, coffee, chocolate drinks (as well as chocolate sweets and biscuits), cola drinks and other fizzy drinks that may contain caffeine.

Take the child to the toilet before bedtime, every single night, even though he continues wetting the bed.

When you go to bed, get him up and take him to the toilet again.

Try to find out from him if there is anything which makes him unhappy about getting up during the night.

Would he rather have a potty in his bedroom, than going to the toilet?

Does he need a low light on in his bedroom through the night?

Does he need a landing light on or a light on in the toilet?

Obviously a waterproof cover should be on the mattress.

Reward System

STAR CHART: The 'star chart' is simple and remarkably effective in some children. Mum or Dad helps the child to draw his own weekly calendar (like the one on the next page). The calendar or chart is kept in a prominent place, for parents and child to see. Every morning that his bed is dry, he is praised and encouraged and is allowed to stick a coloured star on the relevant day. If he is wet no star is put on the chart but do NOT chastise him. Maybe he'll try harder the next night! Once he achieves 3 consecutive dry nights he can stick a GOLD (✷) star on his chart on

79

STAR CHART				
WEEK	1	2	3	4
Monday	✳			
Tuesday				
Wednesday	✳			
Thursday				
Friday	✳			
Saturday	✳			
Sunday	✳			

CHILDREN AND BEDWETTING

* Children who wet the bed are NOT emotionally disturbed.
* Children who wet the bed are NOT deep sleepers.
* Children who wet the bed do NOT have smaller bladders.
* Children who wet the bed are NOT too lazy to get up.
* Children who wet the bed CAN be cured of the problem.

the relevant 3rd night space! Keep the chart going for a month or two and, if all is well, gradually wean him off the idea. If the chart does not produce the desired effect then try the next method.

Alarm Method

Enuresis alarms or buzzers are effective in 80% of children who use them. As with all other interventions, success depends upon the child's and the parent's motivation and determination. These alarms work best when the child does not have to share his bed or bedroom with anyone else.

The alarm is battery operated. With the standard type of alarm a detector mat is placed under the bottom sheet and is connected to a buzzer or alarm at the bedside. The child should be bare from the waist down so that the first drops of urine are detected. When the child starts to wet the bed the urine comes into contact with a sensor which then triggers off the alarm or buzzer. This wakes the child, who can then hold on to his water until he gets to his potty or toilet. Of course he will probably call Mum or Dad, if the alarm hasn't already wakened them, to help and to change him into dry bedding and pyjamas. Success is not instant. Usually the child still wets, but the wet patches

80

The standard alarm system

Mini alarm system

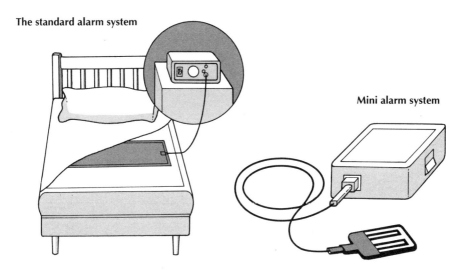

become smaller and smaller, as the child wakens earlier with each alarm!

Basically, the buzzer trains him to waken up when he has a full bladder. Eventually he learns to waken without the buzzer when his bladder feels full. A completely dry bed may not happen until after 2 to 3 weeks of regular use, so do be patient. Before using the alarm let your child become familiar with it and its sound! You don't want the child being terrified by a strange alarm in the middle of the night! A 'mini' enuresis alarm is available (see diagram) which can be worn by the child. The small sensor is fitted inside two pairs of pants and the buzzer is worn on the front of the pyjamas.

Alarms costing from £40 (ex VAT), are available from:
Eastleigh Alarms
(NH Eastwood Ltd)
118 East Barnet Road
Barnet, Herts EN4 8RE

Some health authorities rent or lend them out – find out from your GP or Health Visitor.

Medicines

There are two medications which your GP can prescribe for bed-wetting – *Tofranil* syrup and *Desmospray*, a desmopressin spray.

Tofranil is a treatment which is usually used for depression, but don't be alarmed, your child's bed-wetting is not caused by him being depressed. The reason why this anti-depressant helps with bed-wetting is not fully understood, all we know is that it does work for 85% of bed-wetting children. It should not be used in children under 6 years, and treatment should not continue for longer than 3 months. *Tofranil*, a syrup which is only available on prescription, should be given in the following recommended doses at bedtime:

6 - 7 years – 5ml
8 to 11 years – 5ml to 10ml
over 11 years – 10ml to 15ml

(5ml = 1 teaspoon)

Do not stop the medicine abruptly, but gradually taper off after 2 to 3 months of use. Side effects are not common, but may include dry mouth and constipation.

Desmospray is a nasal spray which works by making the kidneys re-absorb water, so that at night less urine is sent to the bladder. It is only available on prescription. One squirt of the spray is used in each nostril just before bedtime, and the treatment works within 1 hour and lasts for 10 hours. About 70% of children respond to this treatment and, because of its speed of action, it is very useful to prove to a child that they can be dry and they can go on holiday feeling more confident about night dryness.

Best results have been obtained in children over 9 years of age. Side effects are few, and the drug is more expensive than *Tofranil*. It has been found that more children relapse back to bed-wetting on stopping the spray than do on using the alarm system.

So in conclusion – I would recommend as the best method a combination of the alarm system plus star chart.

Helpful organisation
Every parent with a bed-wetting child should contact the following organisation who specialise in advising on this problem. They are tremendously helpful and useful, with some excellent publications for parents and for children:

ERIC
(Enuresis Resource &
Information Centre)
65 St Michael's Hill
Bristol BS2 8DZ

ECZEMA

What is eczema ?

The word eczema comes from a Greek word meaning 'to boil'. What a suitable description! The skin of the eczema sufferer feels hot and itches intensely. Very tiny blisters appear on the skin and it can certainly look as if it is boiling! Irritation of the skin can cause the child to scratch so severely that bleeding occurs. Secondary infection can then set into the skin.

Having probably frightened you with that statement let me now reassure you, at once, that eczema is a condition that responds dramatically well to modern medical treatments. It's a condition that I love to treat because the results are so rewarding both to the doctor and to the worried parent!

Eczema is NOT one single condition. There are many different types of eczema, some producing skin reactions with no obvious cause and other reactions being caused by specific easily recognised external factors. It can affect skin on any part of the body.

DID YOU KNOW THAT THE SKIN IS THE LARGEST ORGAN OF THE BODY?

Eczema produces:
* Redness of the skin.
* Intense itching of the skin.
* Small blisters in the skin.
* Weeping of the skin.
* Dryness and scaling of the skin.

If eczema is allowed to last for a long time without effective treatment the skin can become thickened, discoloured and cracked. Hence it is very important that this distressing condition is treated just as quickly and comprehensively as possible.

Types of eczema
The commonest types of eczema are:
* Atopic eczema
* Seborrhoeic eczema
* Contact eczema
* Pompholyx eczema

The two types that particularly affect babies and children are atopic eczema and seborrhoeic eczema. Contact eczema and pompholyx eczema do occur in children but are more often seen in adults.

ATOPIC (*ay-top-pik*) ECZEMA

This is the most common type of eczema. Often referred to as 'infantile eczema' because it comes on in infancy. Most cases start in the first two years of life. There is often someone else in the family with this condition or with hay fever, asthma or other allergic conditions. These conditions are all closely related, and a child can often be burdened with all three – eczema, hay fever and asthma.

and hand are also affected. The skin looks very inflamed and the child scratches intensely, more often at night, when the skin becomes hot under the bedclothes.

SEBORRHOEIC (*seb-or-ray-ik*) ECZEMA

Seborrhoeic eczema occurs in babies, children and adults. Cradle cap is a type of seborrhoeic eczema of the scalp, often seen during the early months of a baby's life. The skin of the scalp is covered in thick, yellowy, crusty layers. It looks horrific to the mother but rarely troubles the baby!

With seborrhoeic eczema flakiness and redness of the skin is seen on

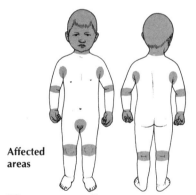

Affected areas

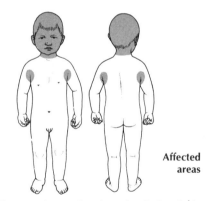

Affected areas

The eczema first appears on the face, scalp and the nappy area. Patches appear in the skin creases on the front of the elbow, front of the wrist, back of the knee joint and around the ankles. The fingers

the neck at the level of the hair line, behind the ears, on the face and even under the armpits. This type of eczema usually clears quickly once treatment is started (see page 89).

84

BY THE WAY, DID YOU KNOW THAT ...

DANDRUFF is a form of seborrhoeic eczema affecting teenagers and adults. It affects the scalp, producing dry scales of skin which flake off, and are shed onto the clothing much to the embarrassment of the sufferer. Often dandruff sufferers have dry skin affecting the eyelids, the crease of skin running from the corner of the nose to the corner of the mouth, behind the ears and even in the ear. This type of dandruff is often resistant to standard shampoos for dandruff, because the skin becomes infected with a type of organism called a fungus or yeast – no, not mushrooms – but a microscopic organism, invisible to the naked eye.

An effective treatment for this resistant type of dandruff, is a substance called ketoconazole. The only shampoo containing this agent is *Nizoral*, and it specifically acts against the offending fungus. This shampoo, cannot be bought over the counter – it is only available on prescription from your GP. When I recommended this on the *This Morning* TV programme we were inundated with letters from people who had cleared their dandruff of 25 years standing within 7 days of using this particular treatment!

CONTACT ECZEMA

In this type of eczema the skin reacts after being in contact with certain substances. The skin becomes reddened, inflamed and itchy at the site of contact with the irritant. A list of the more common agents that cause this type of reaction are listed later under *What causes eczema?* Contact eczema is seen more often in adults than in children.

POMPHOLYX (*pom-foe-liks*) ECZEMA

This is a long-standing and recurring condition which results in tiny blisters affecting the palms of the hands, sides of the fingers and the soles of the feet. As with all eczemas the skin is very itchy. Warm weather commonly provokes this condition and it is often not diagnosed correctly. It is more common in adults than children.

Who gets eczema?

* There are 5 million eczema sufferers in the UK.
* Eczema can run in families – this type is known as atopic eczema.
* If a parent, brother or sister have an allergic-type condition such as eczema, hay fever, asthma or urticaria (heat lumps) there is a 50% chance that any further baby will develop one or more of these conditions.
* Most atopic eczemas appear within the first 2 years of life.
* Fair-skinned babies are more prone to atopic eczema.
* Eczema is more common in children who are NOT breast-fed.
* Eczema is more common in children who are weaned early.
* Eczema is more common in babies who receive cow's milk, eggs or orange juice during their first year.
* Eczema is more common in babies from smoking households.

What causes eczema?

The precise cause of eczema is not fully known. However, we do know that in many patients it is a type of allergic condition in which heredity plays an important role. There is a strong association between eczema, hay fever, asthma, urticaria (heat lumps) and even migraine. If there is a history of these allergic conditions in you or your partner's family your child may be more prone to developing eczema, and therefore precautions should be taken to prevent the condition developing or worsening (see *Can you prevent eczema?* on page 88).

Atopic eczema can be brought on by exposure to cats, dogs or other furry animals. The house dust mite is a common cause of eczema flare-ups. Certain foods can also cause intense reactions in the skin of susceptible children with eczema.

As eczema and all allergic conditions are worse in babies and children exposed to cigarette smoke in the home, it is thought that their sensitive immature immune systems are adversely affected by the chemicals present in tobacco smoke.

Contact eczema is brought on by contact with a substance to which the skin of the sufferer is particularly sensitive. The commonest reactions occur to:

* Nickel – many items of jewellery and metal fasteners on clothing contain nickel. So any reaction in a specific isolated area of skin that has been with a cheaper type of jewellery or a metal zip or clothes' stud will probably be due to contact eczema. Pure gold or silver does not produce this type of eczema, only the cheaper metal alloys.
* Leather in shoes, gloves or watchstraps. The eczema is a reaction of the skin to a chemical called chromate, used in curing leather.
* Cosmetics and perfumes, especially nail-varnish.
* Rubber
* Crease-resistant fabrics. These contain a substance called urea fomaldehyde, which affects some sensitive skins.
* Antihistamine creams can cause marked skin reactions.
* Lanolin can also produce an inflammation in the skin – so beware of creams which contain lanolin in your treatment of eczema. They may make the condition worse rather than curing it.

ECZEMA 'FILE O'FACTS'

* Children with atopic eczema have a dry skin.

* Children with atopic eczema itch more when they are in contact with wool.

* Children with atopic eczema itch more when they sweat.

* 90% of children with atopic eczema are free of the condition before they are 8 years old.

* It's more common in families where there is asthma, hay fever, urticaria and other allergic tendencies.

* Cradle cap usually clears by 2 years of age.

* A child with eczema may be more prone to migraine in later years.

* Eczema is not infectious or contagious and cannot be passed on to close contacts or friends.

Can you prevent eczema?

If there is a genetic tendency for your child to develop eczema because there is a strong family history of this skin complaint, then you cannot completely prevent the disorder from developing. However, you should be able to reduce the severity of the condition, by following these steps:

* If possible fully breast-feed your baby for the first 4–6 months. Do not give the baby any other feed at all, except for water if the weather is hot.

* At 4–6 months wean onto milk-free baby rice, baby vegetables, baby fruits, meat and baby cereals.

* For first 12 MONTHS avoid:
  – cow's milk
  – eggs
  – orange juice
  – ALL wheat products, e.g. bread, cake, biscuits.

* Check the baby food labels for these forbidden items!

* Continue breast feeding, if possible, during baby's first year.

* Avoid coloured or perfumed soaps on child's skin.

* Use only very mild shampoos.

* Avoid creams containing lanolin.

* Avoid biological and low-temperature washing powders.

* Avoid direct wool contact on child's skin.

* Buy pure cotton or cotton-mix clothes. Financial aid may be available – contact your local Social Security office.

* Cotton mittens are available to prevent little ones scratching themselves.

* Avoid clothes with metal fasteners and zips, as baby may develop a contact allergy to metal.

* Do not smoke during pregnancy.

* Try to keep your home free of tobacco smoke.

* Do not allow cats, dogs or any furry animals in the house.

* House dust should be very carefully controlled. (See chapter on Asthma for more information on the house dust mite)

* Avoid certain plants that can produce eczema. Primulas and chrysanthemums are common culprits.

* Be wary of adhesive plasters. *Elastoplast* produce a hypoallergenic plaster.

* If your daughter has very sensitive skin she may have to use cosmetics that are labelled as hypoallergenic, when she reaches teenage years.

* If your child will be having her ears pierced or wearing any jewellery, avoid cheap items. Use only pure gold or silver or heavily plated jewellery. Cheap items contain nickel which causes a bad reaction on the skin.

* Even Mum's nail varnish could cause the child's eczema to flare up!

* As your child gets older you may find that certain foods cause a worsening of the eczema. Potatoes, tomatoes, eggs, milk and products containing milk (read the labels!), wheat-containing foods, cheese and even orange juice are common culprits. In foods, colouring agents, e.g., the orange/red colourant tartrazine, could also affect your child's eczema.

* Certain professions should be avoided by sufferers of eczema because of the possibility of repeated exposure to irritant substances and chemicals. So when your child grows up they should be guided away from hairdressing, nursing, the building industry and garage work.

How should you treat eczema?
Most treatments for eczema are available on prescription from your GP.

Remember that there is NO cure for eczema. In other words no treatment is available that will get rid of eczema permanently. However the condition can most certainly be well controlled with the combined dedication of the parents and the family doctor.

The key to eczema control is:

KEEP THE SKIN SOFT.

PREVENT DRYING-OUT OF THE SKIN.

If the skin is allowed to dry, it becomes itchy. The child then scratches and breaks the skin surface. The skin becomes infected, sore and even more irritating to the child. The skin can be kept soft and drying out of the upper layers of skin can be prevented by the use of emollients.

Emollients
Emollients are mixtures of oils, fats and water which restore the natural, oil balance and moisture content of the skin. They are available as (a) applications such as creams, lotions and ointments, which are rubbed into the skin and as (b) bath liquids.

Advice on use of emollients
Emollients must be used VERY FREQUENTLY and EVERY DAY.

The more often an emollient is applied to the skin the less severe and the less obvious your child's eczema will be. If the eczema is flaring up apply the emollient every hour, if possible! Even if the eczema is under control the emollient should be gently rubbed into the skin 3 times a day. Remember that putting the oils back into the skin will help to prevent the eczema from recurring.

I CANNOT OVER-
EMPHASISE THE
IMPORTANCE OF
FREQUENT DAILY
APPLICATIONS OF
EMOLLIENTS.

Current emollient applications available are as follows:
Alcoderm – cream and lotion
Aquadrate – cream
Dermacare – cream and lotion
Diprobase – cream and ointment
E45 – cream
Eczederm – cream
Humiderm – cream
Hydromol – cream and emulsion
Keri – lotion
Lacticare – lotion
Lipobase – cream

Morhulin – ointment
Natuderm – cream
Oilatum – cream
Sential E – cream
Sudocrem – cream
Ultrabase – cream
Unguentum – cream

All can be bought over the counter and are available on prescription.

Other points to remember:

* Wash your hands before applying the emollient.
* Applying the emollient to your child's skin immediately after bathing aids absorption.
* Gently massage the emollient into your child's skin.
* Emollients are quite safe.
* Your child may respond better to some emollients than others. If one does not work try another, and another until you find one that produces the best effect.
* Some emollients (e.g. *E45* cream) contain lanolin, to which a few eczema sufferers react.
* Get the biggest tub of emollient available. Some are now available in large pump dispensers.

Bath emollients

* Do NOT bathe in water only - this dries out the skin.
* Always add an emollient bath oil to the water.
* Bath emollients currently available are:
  Alpha Keri – contains lanolin
  Aveeno Regular
  Aveeno Oilated
  Balmandol
  Balneum
  Bath E45
  Emulsiderm
  Hydromol
  Oilatum emollient
* Keep your child in the water for 20 MINUTES, if possible. The longer the skin is exposed to the emollient oils the better.
* Beware, the bath will be very slippy!
* Try and avoid using ordinary soaps to cleanse the skin. The chemicals and perfumes they contain can irritate the skin. Two soap substitutes are available over the counter and on prescription:
  Aqueous cream
  Emulsifying ointment
* Pat the skin dry with a soft towel – be gentle.

* After a bath always apply the eczema creams your child is using.

Steroid creams

Steroid creams and ointments reduce the inflammation and the itchiness in eczema. Strengths vary considerably, and ointments are usually better than creams.

Hydrocortisone 1% ointment or cream is safe to use. It can be applied as a twice daily routine treatment. If the eczema is controlled with emollients alone well and good. If not then a steroid ointment or cream such as hydrocortisone 1% should be applied until the skin starts to improve. Hydrocortisone 1% is available without a prescription.

A USEFUL TIP

A bad patch of eczema on a limb can be cleared more quickly, by applying the emollient or steroid ointment and then covering the area with polythene, cut from a plastic bag, or cling-film which is much softer. The ointment will then be completely absorbed into the skin and will not rub off onto clothing or sheets.

If the eczema is severe then a short course of a more effective steroid ointment such as *Modrasone* or *Synalar 1:10* might be prescribed by your doctor.

Antihistamines

Antihistamine creams should NOT be used as they can cause skin reactions. However, certain antihistamine syrups and tablets are very useful in controlling the itch and stopping the itch-scratch-itch cycle.

The older antihistamines can cause marked drowsiness, and this was considered a benefit if the medication was given at night. However, problems arise from inability to get the dosage right, e.g. if insufficient of the antihistamine is given the child can become agitated, hyper-active, restless or irritable - the last thing you want at night in a child already distressed by a skin irritation. If a higher dose is given the child is well sedated but the sedation and drowsiness can persist into the next day, sometimes with a 'hangover' effect, again not to be recommended, especially in a schoolchild.

The new generation of anti-histamines are free from the above side effects and are certainly worth considering (see page 111). They are easy to use, often a once-daily dosage, and they do not cause restlessness or irritability, nor do they usually produce drowsiness or a hangover. They are safe and non-addictive. Contact your GP and he will decide which of these new antihistamines is best for your child as some are not yet recomended for children of a certain age.

Evening primrose oil

The oil of the evening primrose plant has been found to have a beneficial effect on some patients with eczema, though not all. It is more effective in the treatment of atopic eczema but patients don't get an immediate effect and it may have to be taken for 6–8 weeks before any obvious result is seen. In some patients it has had a dramatic effect in improving the eczema.

The preparation called *Epogam* is a capsule which has to be taken orally. It is available on prescription and can also be bought directly from your pharmacist. It is not to be used in children under 1 year of age nor in patients with epilepsy.

The child from 1–12 years should take 2–4 capsules twice daily. Older children should be able to swallow the capsules but for younger ones you should cut the capsules and spread the liquid onto their food, into their drink or even directly into their mouth.

A stronger capsule called *Epogam Paediatric* is available, and this has a lower dose of only 1–2 capsules twice daily.

Summary

* Avoid substances that are known to provoke eczema.
* Use emollient creams/ointments FREELY.
* Bathe regularly using bath emollients.
* Use soap substitutes.
* Steroids – use hydrocortisone 1% as first choice. Then more potent ones to clear skin. Stop these when skin clears.
* Antihistamines – orally, can be useful.
* Consider evening primrose capsules.

Helpful organisation

I highly recommend that eczema sufferers contact the following organisation:

National Eczema Society
Tavistock House East
Tavistock Square
London WC1H 9SR

ASTHMA

Any child that has a persistent cough, more troublesome at night and not responding to cough medicines, may have ASTHMA.

Your child does NOT have to wheeze to have asthma – a cough may be the only symptom.

What is asthma?
Asthma is a condition that affects the tubes that carry air into and through the lungs. These tubes, known as the airways, spread throughout the lungs rather like the branches of a tree. In asthma these tubes are narrowed and this makes breathing more difficult. Narrowing of the airways occurs in three ways.

* Spasm of muscles in the walls of the airways.
* Swelling of the lining of the airways.
* Plugs of sticky phlegm or mucus inside the airways.

All or any of these factors restrict the flow of air in and out of the

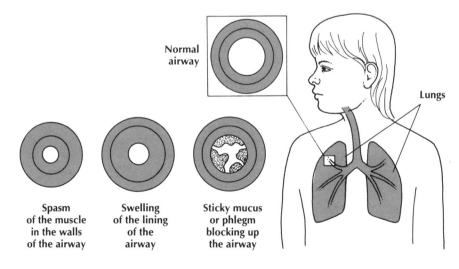

Normal airway

Lungs

Spasm of the muscle in the walls of the airway

Swelling of the lining of the airway

Sticky mucus or phlegm blocking up the airway

94

lungs. Asthma is often best described as trying to breath in and out through a straw! In a fully-fledged attack it is difficult to get your breath, you wheeze a lot and the panic produced by being unable to get your breath makes the condition worse. You cough to try and dislodge the sticky phlegm in the tubes, but the coughing makes you short of breath. Despite the severity of a bad attack, and the fact that asthma cannot be cured, a lot can be done to prevent attacks and many people with asthma lead full normal lives and take part in all sorts of athletic activities. Over half of the children with asthma do grow out of it completely.

Symptoms

If a child has repeated episodes of cough, wheeze and shortness of breath – they have got asthma. The cough is often the most important symptom, because there may be very little wheeze or breathlessness.

The cough comes:
- at night
- on exertion
- when excited
- going out into cold air

Who gets asthma?

* Asthma is more common in young children.

* It affects 1 in 5 children (20%).
* It is twice as common in boys than girls.
* It is more common in families where hay fever, eczema and other allergies are present.
* It is more common in children who had breathing problems at birth (respiratory distress syndrome).
* It is more common in children who had chest infections, such as bronchiolitis, as babies.
* It is more common in children who are exposed to dusty atmospheres, cow's milk and eggs in the first year of life.
* It is less common in breast-fed babies.
* It is more common in the children of smoking parents.
* Asthma can start at any age, though most children who have asthma have had their first attack by the age of 5 years.

Despite effective modern treatments, asthma is on the increase and this is thought to be due to environmental pollution, especially with diesel fumes which make the airways very sensitive to other substances in the atmosphere, such as dust, pollens, etc. About 2,000 deaths occur each year in the UK as a result of asthma.

What causes asthma?

The exact cause of asthma is not known. What we do know is that asthmatics have sensitive or 'twitchy' airways, which react to certain external triggers that set off a tightening or spasm of the airways, along with inflammation of the airtubes and an outpouring of mucus or phlegm.

The triggers that can set off an attack are:

* Infections: especially virus infections such as colds, flu and chest infections.
* Allergies: especially to the house dust mite, pollens and, unfortunately for children, furry pets.
* Exertion: especially exercise such as running and swimming.
* Cold air: especially exerting yourself outside in the cold.
* Feathers: especially in pillows and duvets.
* Excitement: be it nice excitement or bad, such as fear or worry.

* Fumes: such as paint, petrol, pollution and even perfumes.
* Foods: such as peanuts, cold milk, shellfish, strawberries.
* Food colourants such as tartrazine may affect certain people.
* Drugs/medicines: asthmatics young and old should be wary of certain drugs, such as – aspirin, beta-blockers and anti-inflammatory drugs.

How can you prevent asthma?

With asthma more than any other medical condition, prevention is of vital importance. It makes sense to prevent the severe attacks of gasping for breath, as these may not respond to normal treatment measures and can result in emergency hospital admission, or even death!

* Avoid 'trigger' situations. Obviously it is imperative to avoid any situation which you know for certain brings on an attack of asthma. Any one or more of the causes listed above may have to be avoided.

* If there is a history of asthma, hay fever, eczema

or allergies in the family then it would be very wise for a mother to try to breast feed her newborn baby, as this certainly does reduce the chance of allergic diseases in later life.

* Making sure that your child does NOT have any cow's milk for the first 12 months of life is another important step you can take.

* Smoking in pregnancy and after delivery is certainly not to be recommended.

The house dust mite

The commonest cause of asthma is allergy to the house mite, so how do you avoid contact with the house dust mite? In fact, it is not the house dust mite itself to which you are allergic, but the animals faeces or droppings – YUCK! You inhale this little insects' droppings into your lungs and these minute particles trigger off an attack or spasm in the airways.

The house dust mite is a tiny, tiny insect that cannot be seen by the human eye – thank goodness!

It lives in dust anywhere, and loves to feed on the minute scales of human skin that are shed from our bodies. Because the one place where we humans spend a large chunk of time in any 24-hour period is our bed, the house dust mite knows that this is one of the best places for it to take up residence. For the house dust mite the mattress of our bed must seem like heaven. It's warm, dark, comfortable and for 8 hours every day a fresh supply of food showers down upon it, what a des. res.!
There are between 2 and 5 MILLION living mites in your mattress now! Makes you shudder doesn't it? Imagine lying in bed at night when it's gone dark and silent, and right there directly beneath you are millions of these minute monsters munching away on the skin scales that you have shed – it's enough to give us adults nightmares, never mind the little

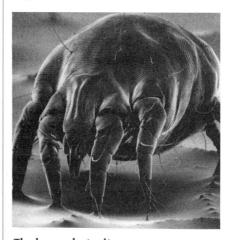

The house dust mite

97

ones! So for goodness sake don't ever tell your children these scary details or show them a picture of the horrendous looking house dust mite, for you'll never get them into the bedroom or bed again!

The mite's droppings are so tiny that they also are invisible to the human eye, but these particles rise in the air and set off an allergic reaction once they are inhaled into the asthmatics lungs.

The house dust mite also lives in pillows, in the carpets, in the curtains, in soft furniture and in all dusty parts of the house.

Control of the house dust mite

Reduce exposure to the house dust mite using the following measures. Total elimination of the house dust mite is impossible. So measures aimed at containing the mite, or reducing it's numbers seem to be more reasonable.

* Do not go around the house with the vacuum cleaner in an attempt to get rid of all the house dust from the carpets, curtains, bedding, mattresses or even off the vinyl or lino floor coverings. 'Hoovering' with a normal domestic appliance, in fact, makes the situation worse! These vacuum cleaners beat the floor and cause vast clouds of house dust mite to be propelled up into the air, ready to be inhaled into the lungs of the poor asthma sufferer. There are special vacuum cleaners for control of house dust and, although they are more expensive, they certainly do appear to work. One of these is *Medivac*. Further information can be obtained from: Medivac, Freepost, Wilmslow, Cheshire SK9 5AA.

* If possible avoid putting carpets on the bedroom floor of the asthmatic child. Use only vinyl or lino, as these can be cleaned using damp cloths to control the dust.

* If there are to be carpets in the bedroom, avoid wool and go for the synthetic materials. The house dust mite isn't keen on synthetic fibres. He's got class - he prefers warm, cosy expensive wool! It has also been shown that synthetic materials develop a static electric charge which holds the dust and

the mite in the carpet, preventing their release into the air and into the lungs!

* Some parents wrap the mattress up in polythene, thus sealing in the house dust mite, and it's droppings. This can be quite effective, but don't forget that the mite also lives in the pillows and the blankets and the duvet. A useful step would be to avoid feather-filled pillows and duvets and go for foam or synthetic materials in pillows, duvets and even mattresses.

* Changing curtains to blinds is another useful step.

* There are two aerosol sprays on the market for use against the house dust mite, one called *Actomite* which seems to have had some success and a new one called *Banamite*. Both will be available from your local pharmacist.

* An effective, though not cheap, method of mite control has come from the bed manufacturers

Slumberland. They have now produced a special cover for the mattress, pillow and duvet made from a material similar to *Gore-tex* the rainproof material. The fine texture of this material is such that the holes between the strands of material are too small for house dust mites and their droppings to get through. The fine holes also prevent human skin scales from entering the mattress and bedding. Further information is available from Slumberland Medicare Ltd, Bee Mill, Shaw Road, Royton, Oldham OL2 6EH.

* Check your child's tubes! Regular assessment of the narrowness of the airways is an important way of preventing severe asthmatic attacks. The patient can actually measure how narrow their airways are by using a simple instrument called the 'peak flow meter'. This is available on NHS prescription, and when used regularly can actually show that the airways are starting to narrow, even

THE
PEAK FLOW METER

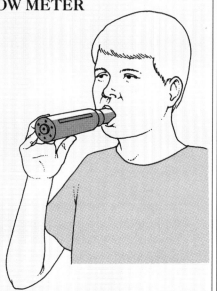

This simple device is held to the mouth, the lips are put over the mouthpiece, and the child blows into the meter as hard and as quickly as he can. The device should be held horizontally during use. If possible 3 measurements should be obtained and the best of three taken as the true reading.

Ideally the child should use the peak flow meter twice a day. When the child is well there will be little difference between the morning and evening readings. If there is more than a 20% difference, then the airways may be narrowing and further treatment may be needed, so do contact your doctor.

All children of 5 years and over should have a peak flow meter at home but children under five usually have difficulty in using the PFM. Regular use of this simple gadget should help prevent severe attacks of asthma.

Read-outs for each age.

Age (years)	Normal Peak Flow	Warning Level
5	170	90
6	190	100
7	210	105
8	230	110
9	250	120
10	280	130
11	300	140
12	330	160
13	350	170
14	380	190
15	410	200
16	430	210

before the patient is aware of any deterioration in their condition.

* One of the most effective ways of preventing asthma attacks is to use the treatment given by your GP, or asthma specialist. Do EXACTLY as you are advised.

How should you treat asthma?
Yourself:
All that you can do is to follow precisely the advice given to you by the doctor regarding your child's asthmatic treatment. There is no place for DIY therapies in the treatment of this potentially serious disease.

GP:
Once your child has been diagnosed as having asthma your GP may well refer him for specialist advice from a chest physician. The treatment for asthma involves the use of medications that are breathed down into the airways to act directly upon the area where the problem exists. So the treatments are administered as inhalers. If the child is able to understand and use the right technique with these inhalers, the treatment proves to be very effective indeed. So much so that most asthmatics with today's

modern medicines can lead normal and often athletic lives.

Adrian Moorhouse, won an Olympic gold medal for Britain in the 1988 Olympic Games in Seoul. He won the 100 metres breaststroke swimming event. He also has asthma! "I was one of the lucky ones," said Adrian, who was diagnosed at the age of 7 years. "If I had not been diagnosed when I was young and given proper treatment, I would never have made it as an Olympic swimmer."

There are three main types of drugs used in the treatment of asthma:

* Bronchodilators – these dilate or open up the airways.
* Anti-allergics – these prevent the airways from narrowing.
* Steroids – these stop inflammation in the airways, reduce phlegm production and reduce the hypersensitivity of the airways.

All are available as inhalers, and there are many different types of inhalers. Some deliver a fine spray, others a fine powder, some are breath actuated, and some are fitted with a whistle to encourage the child to use it the right way!

The BRONCHODILATORS

The most frequently used ones are:

Alupent
Atrovent
Bricanyl
Duovent
Medi-haler iso
Pulmadil
Ventolin

The ANTI-ALLERGICS

Intal
Tilade

The STEROIDS

Becotide 50, 100, 200
Pulmicort

Note: inhaled steroids are very safe and do not produce the side effects sometimes seen with oral steroids. The dose of steroid taken in the inhaled form is very low and can safely be taken over long periods of time.

A typical treatment programme for a child between 5 and 15 years could be as follows:

STEP 1   Start with a bronchodilator, such as *Ventolin* inhaler. 1 puff, 3 to 4 times/day. If not controlled →, step 2.

STEP 2   Add anti-allergic, such as *Intal* inhaler. 1 puff, 4 times/day. Then try to reduce the bronchodilator and keep child free of attacks with regular daily *Intal*. Use *Ventolin* only when child is wheezy. If not controlled →, step 3.

STEP 3   Replace *Intal* with steroid inhaler, such as *Becotide 100*. 1 puff, 2 times/day.

Whatever the combination it is VITAL that the child uses his inhalers every single day. Treatments such as *Intal* and *Becotide* are used to prevent asthma attacks, whereas *Ventolin* helps to prevent but is also very useful in the relieving of the wheeziness that occurs in an asthma attack.

To prevent exercise-induced asthma the child should take 1 or 2 puffs of his *Ventolin* or other

102

bronchodilator 10 minutes before starting his exercise or sport. This simple step could transform your child's life at school and with his playmates. No asthmatic should be classed as an invalid, EXERCISE IS GOOD FOR YOUR CHILD.

Swimming is especially good, because the warm moist air of a swimming-pool causes less irritation to the sensitive airways than the cold dry air in the outside atmosphere.

Your doctor will have given you exact instructions regarding the use of the specific inhaler/inhalers which your child has to use. Follow those instructions to the letter!

Here are some guidelines which may help you in the management of your child's asthma.

* Your child's asthma is a condition which is always present. Even though your child may not be wheezing or coughing the disorder is still there and will flare up if the basic 'twitchiness' and inflammation of the airways is not suppressed on a daily basis. Regular daily treatment keeps the asthma away and keeps your child normal. Asthma needs DAILY treatment – ignore it at your child's peril.

* Before using an inhaler always remember to shake it thoroughly.

* The key to successful asthma control rests in correct inhaler technique. Your child will have to breathe in at exactly the same time that the aerosol inhaler is being squeezed to release its measured amount of medication. This coordination is vital, but is not easy to master. Spacers may help (see below).

* Once the drug is inhaled, the child should hold his breath for 10 seconds to allow the inhaled particles of drug to settle on the walls of the airways deep inside the lungs.

* Spacers: as it is difficult to coordinate the timing of breathing in with the squeezing of the aerosol, it has been found that the use of a spacer makes it easier to administer the

INSTRUCTIONS FOR YOUR CHILD ON HOW TO USE AN AEROSOL INHALER PROPERLY

(These instructions are reproduced from *How To Cope With an Asthma Attack,*
a booklet published by National Asthma Campaign)

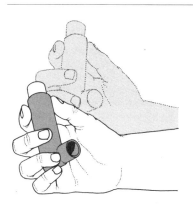

Step 2: Holding the inhaler as shown, breathe out gently (but not fully) and then immediately ...

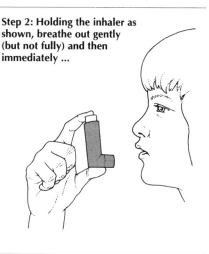

Step 1: Remove the cover from the mouthpiece, and shake the inhaler vigorously.

Step 3: Place the mouthpiece in the mouth and close your lips around it.

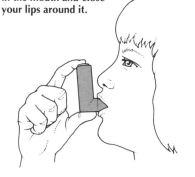

Step 4: After starting to breathe in slowly and deeply through your mouth, press the inhaler firmly to release the medication and continue to breathe in.

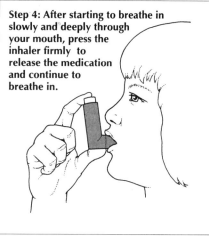

Step 5: Hold your breath for 10 seconds, or as long as is comfortable, before breathing out slowly.

Step 6: If you are to take a second inhalation you should wait at least one minute before repeating Steps 1 to 5.

N.B. After use replace the cover on the mouthpiece.

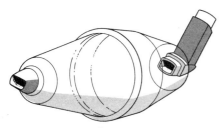

How a spacer works

treatment and to get the drug down into the lungs at the right dose.

The inhaler is fitted into one end of the spacer. It is squeezed and the dose of the drug is delivered as a fine mist into the body of the spacer. The child then, in his own time, takes several breaths through the mouthpiece of the spacer, receiving the medication without any problems. For babies a make-shift spacer can be made from a disposable plastic or polystyrene cup.

Two main types of spacer are available on NHS prescription:

Volumatic – for *Ventolin and Becotide.*
Nebuhaler – for *Bricanyl and Pulmicort.*

Antihistamines

Many children have warning signs before an attack starts. Some have sneezing bouts, runny noses or a tickly cough and if one reacts quickly enough with treatment the attack may well be prevented.

The use of antihistamines in tablet or medicine form can be useful in this situation to ward off an attack. In fact, it is surprising that since antihistamines are effective in allergic conditions they seem to be under-used in the treatment of asthma – the main cause of which is an allergic reaction in the small airways.

This may be due to the fact that the older antihistamines caused all sorts of problems such as drowsiness and, in children, irritability. This is certainly not the case these days with the new generation of antihistamines which are more user-friendly in that they need to be taken only once daily and do not now cause drowsiness or irritability (see page 111/112).

Ask your GP for his advice, as some are not yet recommended for children under a certain age.

Helpful organisation

The National Asthma Campaign (The Junior Asthma Club) 300 Upper Street London N1 2XX Asthma helpline: 0345 010203

105

HAY FEVER

What is hay fever?

Hay fever – what a misleading name. The condition is not caused by hay, nor does the patient get a fever!

Hay fever is an allergic reaction to pollens in the air. When the nose is affected by an allergic condition the disorder is known as allergic rhinitis. When the allergy occurs only at certain times of the year, as hay fever does, the disorder is called seasonal allergic rhinitis. Some children are not allergic to pollen but to other substances such as the house dust mite, which is present all year round – then the condition is known as perennial allergic rhinitis.

Pollen particles are very tiny grains, invisible to the human eye, shed by plants into the air. The symptoms come on only at certain times of the year, and the rest of the year the child is totally free of all symptoms.

The commonest symptom is an irritation inside the nose which causes the child to sneeze and suffer from a runny nose that often becomes blocked, making breathing through the nose very difficult. As pollen hits the eyes there follows an itchiness of the skin inside the upper and lower eyelids, along with a redness and reflex watering of the eyes. The child often feels a tickly irritation affecting the palate and the back of the throat. As pollen enters the tubes going down to the lungs the allergic reaction there can cause a narrowing of the airways. A wheezy sound and sensation is experienced and a full blown asthma attack can follow in susceptible individuals.

Overall, it's a very unpleasant experience to suffer for a child during the spring and summer months, when all his friends are playing outside totally unhindered. Well, there's no need for your child to suffer! (See the section on treatment that follows.)

Symptoms
* Itchy eyes.
* Red streaming eyes.

* Itchy nose and throat.
* Runny nose.
* Sneezing.
* Wheezy chest.
* Muzzy head.

If you think your child is always getting colds or is prone to persistent catarrh, think again, for he may have hay fever. If he often rubs his eyes, and his nose runs with a clear mucus (rather than a yellow or green mucus) then talk to your GP, who will help in establishing the diagnosis. Pollens are put out into the air, not just by flowers but also by trees and grasses. Some people get hay fever symptoms from moulds and spores in the air from fungi. Hay fever sufferers are not allergic to all pollens, but to the pollen of a specific flower, or tree or grass. They develop their allergic reaction at the point where pollen grains come into contact with the sensitive membranes of the body, such as eyes, nose, throat, lungs and ears.

Urban hay fever
Hay fever and allergies in general are on the increase. This is thought to be due to an increase in the level of pollution in the atmosphere. In cities, diesel fumes and the gas nitrogen dioxide from polluted air are thought to effect the sensitive mucous membranes in such a way that their defence mechanisms over-react in an abnormal way to pollen grains, fungal spores and moulds. It has also been suggested that the 'greenhouse' effect is making winters milder, and summers longer and warmer, so that more pollen is produced over a longer period of time. Ozone, which is also on the increase in certain areas, is thought to affect the body's allergic response mechanism in a similar way to diesel and nitrogen dioxide.

The end result of all these effects is that we are now seeing an increase in hay fever symptoms and sufferers in city dwellers despite a DROP in the pollen count! In the olden days hay fever sufferers wouldn't dare venture into the countryside because of exposure to higher levels of pollen, from trees and grasses. Now, however, we find ourselves in a totally reversed situation where the city dweller may be better off escaping the city fumes to alleviate his urban hay fever!

City cyclists wearing masks to avoid diesel, nitrogen dioxide and ozone are wasting their time unless their masks are air-tight and contain charcoal filters.

The hay fever season
TREES: Pollen grains from trees

107

HAY FEVER 'FILE O' FACTS'

Those most likely to develop hay fever are:

* Those born between January and June, inclusive.
* Those born to mothers who smoked during their pregnancy.
* Those born to mothers who continued smoking during the child's infancy and early childhood.
* Those who are bottle-fed.
* Those who are fed cow's milk during their first 12 months of life.
* Boys more than girls.
* Those children who are the older ones in a family.
* Those who already have hay fever in the family.
* Those who have asthma, eczema or other allergies in the family.
* Those who have other allergic conditions themselves, such as asthma and eczema.
* And would you believe it? One team of researchers has found that hay fever is more common in shy people!

such as hazel, elm and yew are present in the atmosphere as early as February and March. So a child who is allergic to those pollens will start with symptoms early in the year, though the symptoms due to tree pollen allergy are not as bad as flower or grass pollen allergies.

GRASSES: There are many different types of grass, but most of them disperse their pollens from May to August, the peak time being in June and July. It's at this time of the year that most hay fever sufferers are at their worst – typical isn't it – just the time when older children and students are taking examinations that may affect the rest of their lives! It's very difficult to study or concentrate with persistent sneezing bouts, runny itchy eyes, a runny nose and gasping for breath!

FUNGI & WEEDS: A child getting hay fever symptoms in late August and in September will probably be allergic to spores released from fungi, such as the aspergillus mould, or from pollen released by nettles and dock plants.

Who gets hay fever?
It can come at any age, thought it is unusual to see it in the under 5s.

At least 10 to 15% of the population

get hay fever at some time, and certainly 20% of teenagers suffer from the condition. It's rare to see hay fever in an old-age pensioner, it must be due to the fact that as we all get older we seem to dry up and dry out, and conditions such as runny eyes and runny noses seem to disappear.

What causes hay fever?

Pollen! No more, no less! Though having said that, pollen grains have been around for thousands of years (they have been discovered in the wrapping materials of Egyptian mummies) and yet hay fever was very rare 100 years ago! It certainly seems that the condition has got worse since the Industrial Revolution, thus giving more credence to the connection between increased pollution and an increasing incidence of hay fever (see urban hay fever above), and many other allergic conditions! This allergic reaction of modern-day man, in the lining of the nose, eyes, throat, ears and airways, is an over-reaction of the body's defence mechanism caused by exposure to pollen grains in the air.

Can you prevent hay fever?

The only way your child can prevent hay fever is to reduce his contact with pollen. This can be done by protecting the eyes, nose and throat by keeping the house windows closed in early morning and late evening (and night-time) when the pollen grain population is more numerous. Hot air in the late morning and early afternoon rises from ground level up into the atmosphere, carrying with it most of the pollen. As the air cools in the late afternoon, the cool air descends, bringing the pollen down with it.

When your child is out in the car keep the car windows closed.

If possible, the wearing of sunglasses when out can prevent a lot of pollen from directly entering into the eyes.

Keep your eye on the pollen count. When it is high, avoid parks, gardens, and the open spaces – if you can!

Holidays can be ruined by hay fever symptoms, so if your child suffers badly with hay fever holidays by the seaside are best, followed by holidays in high mountainous regions where there may be some pollen, though not a lot.

Some people are helped by the use of ionisers in the home, although there is some controversy over whether these really do work.

109

One houseplant in particular can cause symptoms of hay fever at any time of the year, and also symptoms of asthma. The plant is the Weeping Fig, which is a very popular house plant. One species of the weeping fig, called ficus benjamina is especially likely to cause an allergic reaction So check to see if you have this plant in your house, and if you have I would advise that you get rid of it, just to be sure that your child is not being exposed to yet another factor which might cause a flare up of his hay fever or more seriously his asthma.

How should you treat hay fever?
To obtain the best results every child with hay fever should commence their treatment BEFORE their symptoms are

DID YOU KNOW?

People with hay fever and asthma are prone to swellings inside the nose, called nasal polyps, which can block one or both nostrils.

People with hay fever and asthma may not know they have nasal polyps but will be highly prone to an allergy to aspirin, tartrazine (the orange-yellow food colourant, number E102) and other colouring agents known as the azo dyes.

Because the allergic reaction to aspirin itself can be so serious I would advise that:

ANY PERSON WHO HAS BOTH
HAY FEVER AND ASTHMA
SHOULD AVOID ASPIRIN.

This applies more to children over the age of 12 years as aspirin should not be given to any child under 12 because it has been linked with a condition called Reye's syndrome, a serious disorder.

expected to start. If your child has hay fever you will know after one or two seasons when he is at his worst and you will have a good idea when the problem usually starts. As most hay fever sufferers are starting to get symptoms in late May and early June, the best advice I can give is:

Start treating hay fever in LATE APRIL even if the symptoms have not appeared and continue THROUGHOUT the hay fever season.

Yourself:

Antihistamines are the first choice treatment for hay fever. Antihistamines are effective at relieving the eye symptoms, the runny nose, the itchy nose, the sneezing and the itchy palate. They are less effective at relieving the nasal congestion.

There are many antihistamines which you can buy over the counter at your local chemist's shop, and the pharmacist will advise you accordingly. Here is a list of some that are available and can be used in children:

* *Aller-eze*
* *Hismanal* (over 12s only)
* *Dimotane Plus*
* *Optimine*

* *Periactin*
* *Phenergan*
* *Piriton*
* *Pollon-eze* (over 12s only)
* *Seldane* (over 12s only)
* *Sudafed Plus*
* *Tavegil*
* *Triludan*

Many of these can cause sedation and drowsiness. If you want to avoid that, the new generation antihistamines which do not cause drowsiness should be used. These are *Hismanal, Pollon-eze* and *Seldane*. All have the added advantage that they need only be given once a day, but are only suitable for the over 12s. *Triludan* is also non-sedating, and can be used in children over 6 years, but is recommended at a twice-daily dosage.

So read the instructions on the bottle very carefully, paying particular attention to the dosage recommended for the age of your child.

As advised above, start the treatment before symptoms commence and continue throughout the season. If your child is not kept symptom free, go to see your GP for additional items of treatment, which are only available on prescription.

GP:

ANTIHISTAMINES: Because antihistamines are always the first choice of treatment, I should let you know of some of the other antihistamines which your GP may prescribe for hay fever. Many of those listed above are available on prescription, which will not therefore cost you anything for children under the age of 16 years!

The new generation antihistamines for children over 12 years, and which do not cause drowsiness available on prescription are:

* *Clarityn*
* *Hismanal*
* *Semprex*
* *Triludan*
* *Triludan Forte*
* *Zirtek*

Clarityn, Triludan Forte and *Zirtek* are all one-a-day, and quick acting. *Hismanal* is once daily, but takes several days to achieve its full effect.

NASAL SPRAYS/DROPS: There are 3 types of nasal spray or nasal drop treatment available:

* Steroids.
* Anti-allergy sprays.
* Decongestants.

Steroid Sprays/Drops. Do not be put off by the word 'steroid'. These sprays deliver a very tiny dose of a steroid into the nostrils, where the drug acts very effectively in stopping the inflammation, nasal irritation and runny nose. The drug is not absorbed into the body, it is safe to use and does NOT produce any dangerous steroid effects in the body. They should be used without any worry as they are so effective in virtually eliminating the symptoms of hay fever.

The sprays/drops available are:

* *Beconase*
* *Betnesol*
* *Dexa-rhinaspray*
* *Rhinocort*
* *Syntaris*
* *Vista-methasone.*

None of these should be used in children under the age of 6 years. *Beconase* aqueous nasal spray and *Syntaris* are popular, because they need only be used twice a day, morning and evening.

Anti-allergy sprays/drops. These are used more to prevent the allergic reaction in the nose, and unfortunately have to be used 4–6 times a day, and are not as effective as the steroid sprays in eliminating hay fever symptoms. There is only one brand on the

HAY FEVER ... MY WAY

I find the most helpful and simple combination of treatments for children over the age of 6 years is:

BECONASE AQUEOUS NASAL SPRAY

Two squirts into each nostril, morning and evening.

PLUS

TRILUDAN SUSPENSION

One teaspoon (5ml), morning and evening.

Half a Triludan tablet, twice daily, can be given if the suspension is not suitable.

Obviously your own GP will have his own method of treating the condition, so don't go forcing my ideas upon him! Be diplomatic.

market but it is available in several different delivery systems:

* *Rynacrom* nasal spray
* *Rynacrom* nasal drops
* *Rynacrom* cartridges
* *Rynacrom* compound spray.

Decongestants. As these act only temporarily and should not be used on regular basis long term, I would not recommend them in the treatment of hay fever.

EYE DROPS The only drops that I would use in the treatment of the eye symptoms in hay fever are:

* *Opticrom*

For adults or children the dose is 1 or 2 drops in each eye four times a day. These drops should not be used in any patient wearing soft contact lenses. In most cases of hay fever the eye symptoms are controlled by the antihistamine tablets or syrup. If they are not then the use of *Opticrom* as early in the season as possible is to be recommended.

EXAMINATION TIME If the above suggested treatments do not work and the hay fever is severe, at an important time in an older child's life such as GCSE, A–level or college/university examination time, the patient could be helped by an injection of a long acting steroid.

The decision to give this rests solely with your GP. But two steroids that have been used in these exceptional situations are:

* *Depo-medrone* injection
* *Kenalog* injection.

Sometimes a course of oral steroid tablets will be given instead to get the student through such a difficult time. None of these steroid injections or tablets will be given for a long period of time – they are short-term measures.

Helpful organisation

The British Allergy Foundation
St Bartholomew's Hospital
West Smithfield
London EC1A 7BE

SMOKING
AND YOUR BABY

ACTIVE AND PASSIVE SMOKING

About one third of the adult population smoke. Most of these adult smokers know that smoking is not good for their health, and yet they continue to smoke. Well that's their decision and fair enough it's their health! However, if someone else's smoking is shown to cause damage to another person's health and that other person is a non-smoker then the situation changes completely. A person who has chosen not to smoke should not be exposed to cigarette smoke as there is now very impressive evidence that non-smokers face real risks of damage to their health from other people's smoke.

The inhalation of smoke into the body when a smoker smokes a cigarette is ACTIVE smoking. The inhalation of smoke from someone else's cigarette by a non-smoker is PASSIVE smoking. This is also known as involuntary smoking, second-hand smoke or environmental tobacco smoke (ETS).

Tobacco smoke in the air contains cancer-causing particles and many other toxic chemicals which are known to cause disease in non-smokers who have no other option but to breathe those substances into their bodies from the air in their immediate environment.

CIGARETTE SMOKE AND THE UNBORN BABY

* Every day a pregnant smoker takes into her body 200 shots of nicotine and thousands of other chemicals in tobacco smoke.

* From the moment of conception a smoking mother's bloodstream delivers those chemicals directly to the cells of her developing baby.

* As every cell grows in the developing baby – to produce its fingers, arms, toes, legs, face, brain, heart and internal organs – it is

115

SMOKING 'FILE O'FACTS'

* Tobacco smoke contains 4000 chemicals.
* The three major substances are nicotine, tar and carbon monoxide.
* Nicotine is as addictive as heroin - that's why many smokers find it extremely difficult to give up smoking.
* Nicotine reaches the brain within seven seconds of inhaling the smoke. That's faster than an intravenous injection, which would take 14 seconds to reach the brain!
* Nicotine is a very quick-acting tranquilliser – it relaxes you.
* Nicotine can also act as a stimulant – giving you a 'lift'.
* The average smoker consumes 20 cigarettes per day.
* Whilst smoking a cigarette ten puffs of smoke are inhaled.
* A 20-a-day smoker takes 200 puffs of smoke into their body each day.
* A smoker, therefore, takes 200 shots of nicotine into their brain every single day!
* In one year, the average smoker puts 73,000 shots of addictive nicotine into their brain – no wonder it's difficult to quit smoking!
* As well as nicotine, a smoker is receiving 200 shots of tar, carbon monoxide and 3,997 other chemicals every day!

exposed each day to 200 shots of a mixture of 4,000 chemicals.

* The unborn baby is being exposed to the effects of passive smoking. It has no choice in the matter -- it can't escape from exposure to these chemicals– it can't leave the womb!

* Even BEFORE the baby is born he has already received 56,000 SHOTS.

* No wonder the babies of smoking mothers are prone to all sorts of medical problems.

THE EFFECTS OF PASSIVE SMOKING ON THE CHILD

The following disorders affect the babies of both non-smoking mothers and smoking mothers but the sad fact is that ALL these conditions occur more commonly in children whose mothers smoke.

* Miscarriage
* Stillbirth
* Premature delivery
* Death in the first month of life
* Physical deformities, e.g. cleft palate or harelip.
* Abnormalities of the nervous system
* Cot death
* Immaturity both mental and physical
* Childhood cancers – leukaemia and Hodgkin's disease
* Meningitis
* Deafness from glue ear
* Poorer progress in school
* Asthma
* Pneumonia and chest infections
* Allergies

This is not meant to be a comprehensive list, it is only a list of SOME of the risks that babies face when their mothers smoke!

Ideally, a woman should stop smoking well before she becomes pregnant. Giving up cigarettes is not easy – I know, I have run stop-smoking programmes for 15 years and in as many countries. I know the problems and difficulties (see page 144)!

If you are pregnant, and find it impossible to give up, I would strongly recommend that you drastically cut down on your daily cigarette consumption. Better that you only have five per day, (one after each meal and two for when you're desperate!), than continue smoking 20 cigarettes every day throughout your pregnancy.

However, after delivery, your little baby is still going to be exposed to the effects of passive smoking. If you have played Russian roulette with your baby's health by smoking through pregnancy, and been lucky, now look at how delicate and beautiful your newborn baby is. Subjecting him to passive smoking from your cigarettes, and your partner's if he smokes, perpetuates many of the dangers mentioned previously.

If you can't stop smoking for your own sake, do it for your child. Give your baby the best start in life – GOOD HEALTH.

117

THE NASTIES

HEADLICE AND NITS

> **WARNING!**
> I bet you can't get through this section without scratching your head!

What are headlice and nits?
Headlice are tiny insects about 2mm long. They are parasites which live on the head and feed by sucking blood from the scalp. As the insect pierces the skin to drink its next meal of blood an irritation is felt and the child scratches his head.

With hundreds of headlice feeding throughout day and night you can see why the poor child is repeatedly itching his scalp!

The headlice lay their eggs on the hairs, usually at night, when the child is still. Nits is the name given to the eggs, not the lice. The word for a single insect is a 'headlouse' or 'louse'.

THE LOUSY LIFE OF A LOUSE!

The nits, or eggs, are tiny brownish oval-shaped objects, which are glued to individual hair shafts, near to the scalp, where it is warm. Each female louse, lays 6 to 9 eggs each night. Female headlice out number the males 4 to 1, and the female will mate after laying each single egg. The egg takes 8 days to hatch, and after that the baby louse emerges, 'gnashers at the ready'. The now-empty shell case, or nit, appears more white in colour but still adheres to the hair shaft. It is this empty shell that is detected, for it is more easily seen than the unhatched, live egg. The hungry baby louse now bites into the skin of the scalp for his first feed of human blood! He then feeds 5 times a day, grows, reaches adulthood at 10 days, takes an interest in all those female lice (he's outnumbered 4 to 1) and starts mating to produce more lice.

A headlouse likes to travel, not only around the head he is on, but also onto other heads – he wants to see the world – unfortunately for close friends of the poor child with active infestation! So he and his mates travel from head to head, leaving trails of havoc behind them. After such a hectic life the headlouse reaches the end of his lifespan at about 5–6 weeks.

REMEMBER – DO NOT REACT WITH HORROR IF YOUR CHILD HAS HEADLICE. YOUR FEAR WILL ALSO ALARM YOUR CHILD.

Who gets headlice?

Anyone in contact with another person who has headlice can easily pick up the condition, no matter how clean you are or how frequently you bathe or wash your child's hair.

Lice love any head, clean or dirty, all they want is blood, and hair to lay eggs on! Obviously, therefore, young girls with long hair are particularly at risk.

When children are found to have nits it is presumed that they have caught the headlice from someone at school. This is often NOT the case! Brief head-to-head contact is not enough to spread the majority of headlice, because it is now considered that closer, longer contact is the obvious mode of transmission of the louse. This situation happens more often with adult to child contact, and if a child is getting repeated infestations you should look at your child's close adult contacts.

An older person may have quite bad headlice infestation without any symptoms, and this happens more often in older women. More often than not it is these long-term headlice carriers that keep passing it back to children.

An example of this happened in a little village near to Cambridge where the school children were getting repeated headlice infestation, despite treatment.

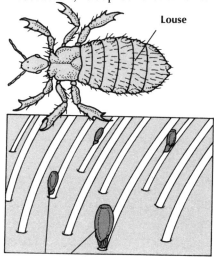

Louse

Nits on hair shafts

119

Apparently the children frequently popped into the local corner shop on their way from school, and the owner, a little old lady, was in the habit of picking up the children, sitting them on the counter, and giving them a biscuit and a cuddle. She was unaware of her own headlice, and so the children got more than their biscuit and cuddle!

Can you prevent headlice?
You can't do anything that will definitely prevent your child from getting headlice.

Washing the child's hair, keeping it short or whatever other steps you might want to take will not prevent the headlouse from hopping onto your child's head from another

HEADLICE
'FILE O' FACTS'

* Headlice lay their eggs on the hair close to the skin.
* Hair grows at $^1/_2$ inch per month.
* On discovering nits in your child, measure distance from scalp to nit.
* This tells you how long your child has been infested with these headlice, e.g. nits 1 inch from the scalp tell you that your child has had the lice for about two months!
* The average time of discovery in schools is 4 months after the child has caught them.
* Itching often does not appear until the child has had the lice for a couple of months.
* After 2 months there could be 150–200 lice living on the head.
* It is estimated that 1 in 10 primary school children have headlice.
* The Isle of Man is totally free of lice, following a 'bug-busting' purge in 1986.
* Headlice can and do develop resistance to various anti-lice shampoos and treatments. If your child is not responding to treatment discuss this with your school nurse, health visitor or GP. They may know what the local Health Authority's advice is on current effective treatment.

infested person. The best way of preventing spread to unaffected members of the same family is to treat the child promptly and CORRECTLY, and also to treat all other members of the family at the same time. Re-infestation is prevented by repeating the treatment 1 week after the initial treatment – see below.

How should you treat headlice?
Yourself:
As soon as you get over the horror and unnecessary feelings of shame that hit you when you discover that your child has caught headlice you will probably run at full pelt down to the chemist. There are some very effective treatments available, but you should bear in mind that the effectiveness of any treatment depends upon the concentration of the preparation used and the length of time it remains in contact with the scalp.

Shampoos become diluted with water and are not in contact with the scalp long enough to give a 100% success rate, so I would recommend that you try LOTIONS rather than shampoos. When using a lotion, keep the bathroom window open as these are very strong smelling chemicals. Take special care with a child who has asthma. If your child has eczema of the scalp, or inflamed skin on the scalp as a result of scratching, then use an aqueous (water) based lotion rather than an alcohol (spirit) based lotion, which might sting the affected skin.

All treatments for headlice are available over the counter from your local chemist.

The following lotions are recommended:

* *Derbac-M* (aqueous)
* *Prioderm* (alcohol)
* *Suleo-M* (alcohol)

These lotions should be applied liberally to DRY hair, and then left on overnight for 12 hours. Shampoo off the next morning with your normal shampoo, rinse, and then comb through with a fine-toothed 'nit comb' whilst the hair is wet. Many of the treatments come with a nit comb, which is so fine toothed that it dislodges the nits from the hairs. The process of combing the hair must be done slowly and methodically. To make combing of the wet hair easier, I would recommend that you apply some hair conditioner after rinsing out the shampoo.

REPEAT this procedure one week later.

ALL MEMBERS OF THE FAMILY, HOUSEHOLD AND CLOSE CONTACTS MUST BE TREATED AT THE SAME TIME, NOT FORGETTING GRANDPARENTS!
(Remember the old lady in the village shop!).

The school should also be notified, so swallow your pride and don't be ashamed to tell the teacher. All children should then be checked by the school nurse, or all the children in the same class should be treated, as well as their families.

Ideally the whole school and all their family members should receive treatment at the same time, but can you imagine the difficulties that arise from trying to organise that mammoth task? This is the only way to tackle the problem of headlice infestation throughout the community.

If the headlice are not cleared with the above lotions it may be that they have developed resistance to the treatment you are using. If this has happened contact your local school nurse or health visitor who will advise you on the current regulations for your particular area.

Other treatments that have also been found to be effective are:

* *Full Marks*
* *Lyclear*
* *Carylderm*
* *Clinicide*
* *Derbac-C*
* *Suleo-C*

One treatment that is not recommended for headlice is a shampoo called *Quellada Application PC*. This shampoo, which might possibly be offered to you by the chemist, contains a chemical called lindane which has been reported to cause convulsions in children and adults.

With headlice, there is no point in fumigating the house or bedroom, or clothing. Headlice need human blood to live, they cannot live on carpets, or furnishings. Their eggs only exist on hairs so I would suggest that you wash pillow cases, brushes, combs, and any other articles that may have lots of hair strands on them. Do this at the same time as treatment is being administered to everyone in the household. Don't be too obsessional about this, concentrate more on treating the scalp of all affected persons and all household members at the same time, and again one week later.

Many authorities recommend a rotating programme using a different preparation every 6 months to prevent the headlice becoming resistant to treatment. They'd be better off attacking the problem in one fell swoop by treating every single child and adult in their locality on the same day – in other words going for a 'bug-busting' day, as the Isle of Man did in 1986!

WARTS

What are warts?

Warts are small, brown swellings on the skin. They are usually present on the hands and feet and sometimes on the neck, armpits or even the face. In adults they also affect the genital areas. Notice, they do not occur on parts of the body where the hands can't reach too easily. They are spread by contact with other warts or other people with warts. Warts in children, though looking unsightly, are not serious and are usually painless unless one grows under a nail, or on the sole of the foot.

A wart that grows on the sole of the foot is known as a verruca (*ver-rook-ah*), or plantar wart, and when there are several they are called verrucae (*ver-rook-ay*) not verrucas! If you

are unsure about a swelling on your child's skin make an appointment to see your GP, who will then be able to make an exact diagnosis and put your mind at rest.

Who gets warts?

About 10% of the population have warts. Warts are passed on by coming into contact with other people who have warts.

For example, a verruca on the sole of the foot can only be picked up by coming into contact with the virus that causes warts. The commonest situation for this to happen is in public swimming pools, paddling pools and showers. People with a verruca will shed the virus from the verruca on their foot, as they stand in the showers or as they stand by the side of the swimming pool. An innocent 'victim' picks up the virus on the sole of their foot and, bingo, they've got themselves a nasty little verruca sdeveloping on their foot.

Warts on the hands commonly spread from one finger to another by direct contact. These are often termed 'kissing warts' in that they have spread by direct kissing of the skin surface with another.

What causes warts?

Warts arise frequently on areas of skin where the skin is subject to

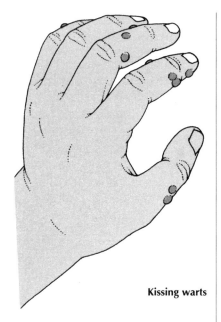

Kissing warts

repeated trauma such as the soles of the feet, hands and children's knees. Warts near fingernails are often spread from one finger to another by the child biting its nails!

Can you prevent warts?

The only way to prevent the spread of warts and verrucae is for sufferers to have active treatment of their warts and not to use public swimming areas without wearing a 'verruca sock', which is a thin plastic, close-fitting sock made from similar material used in swimming hats. These verruca socks can be obtained from your local pharmacist or the manufacturers, Plastsoks, Carita House, Stapely, Nantwich,

Cheshire. Children who do not have verrucae cannot do anything active themselves to avoid picking up the virus, unless they themselves want to wear plastic socks to prevent their own feet coming into contact with swimming pool surfaces.

Some local authorities ban children with plastic verruca socks from swimming in their pools - this is a totally ridiculous attitude to take, for all the child needs to do is NOT to wear their plastic sock. They can use the pool and secretly infect everybody in the public baths!

As long as a child with a verruca wears a plastic verruca sock there is NO reason why they should be banned from using public swimming pools.

How should you treat warts and verrucae?
Yourself:
Don't look upon warts as horrific ugly defects upon your child's skin. Remember your child may be very sensitive about his warts as he may well have had a lot of nasty comments from his friends at school – children can be very cruel to one another! Reassure your child that these warts will go away, but they may be slow to respond. They are not serious, nor are they dangerous.

124

WARTS 'FILE O'FACTS'

* 70% of warts disappear on their own within 2 years.

* Warts are caused by a virus – the human papilloma virus.

* Warts are passed on by contact (direct or indirect) with other warts.

* Expect 2–3 months of DIY treatment to clear the warts.

On finding a wart or a verruca, check to see if your child has any more elsewhere.

Leave the wart alone – most clear up without any treatment.

If you do want to treat the wart yourself there are several wart treatments obtainable from your pharmacist. Here are some of the more popular ones:

All Warts:
* *Callusolve*
* *Cuplex*
* *Duofilm*
* *Glutarol*

* *Novaruca*
* *Salactol*
* *Salactac*
* *Verucasep*

Verrucae only:
* *Posalfilin*
* *Verucur*
* *Verrugon*

NONE of the above should be used on warts that are present on the face or genital region.

These should be referred to your GP who will recommend specialist advice.

With all of the above treatments follow the instructions on the container very, very carefully. These liquids are powerful, and may burn or badly sting normal skin if the liquid is carelessly applied beyond the surface of the wart or verruca itself. Remember that treatment may take a while to have its effect, so do be patient.

GP:

If the above treatments have no effect, the GP may refer your child to a skin specialist (dermatologist). Do not be surprised if there is a long wait before your child is seen. Warts are very common, so there are lots of children with them, and lots of children on waiting lists to

125

see specialists. After being seen your child may have a further wait before receiving treatment. Skin specialists know that 80% of warts clear on their own without any treatment whatsoever. So many children on waiting lists find that by the time they are sent for their warts have actually cleared up! There's sometimes a reason for a long waiting list!

If your child receives treatment from a specialist, it will usually involve freezing the wart with liquid nitrogen. The freezing of the wart actually kills the virus in the wart and the wart drops off some time later, or can be quite simply removed at a later date. Sometimes the wart may have to be removed surgically or cauterized by the specialist.

WORMS

What are worms?
Worms are parasites that live in the intestines or bowels. The most common type of worm encountered in the UK is the threadworm. The worms are passed in the stools and they actually look like pieces of fine white thread, crawling over the surface of the child's faeces. The child often complains of an itchy bottom, particularly at night.

This is due to the female threadworm coming out of the intestine to lay her eggs at night, outside the anus. She will lay about 10,000 eggs at the opening of the back passage and this causes intense irritation for the poor child.

DO NOT show your child the worms, NOR should you tell him that he has worms, as that could cause him all sorts of worry.

To a child, 'worms' are earthworms and the thought of those creatures crawling around inside the tummy are quite horrific!

Threadworms do not cause any serious problems and are easily eliminated.

Symptoms

* Itchy bottom, especially at night.

* Disturbed sleep.

* Irritability and restlessness.

* Itchy vagina, in girls, maybe with a slight discharge.

* Sometimes in children abdominal pain may occur.

Who gets threadworms?

Quite simply anybody who has been in contact with someone who has worms, or who has eaten uncooked food, such as salad, handled by an infected person, who has not washed their hands thoroughly after being to the toilet! Quite scary really, isn't it?

Girls are more prone to threadworms than boys.

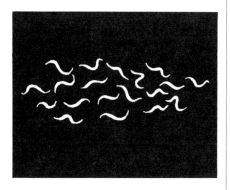

Threadworms appear at night and look just like small pieces of white thread at the entrance to the anus.

What causes threadworms?

Threadworm eggs are passed from an infected person onto an uninfected individual. The eggs enter the body via the mouth, through food or hand to mouth transfer. When the egg is swallowed it develops inside the intestine to recommence a whole new life cycle.

Can you prevent threadworms?

Prevention is best achieved by taking the following steps:

* Adequately treat all the family members of a child with threadworms.

* All members of a family with threadworms, should make sure that their nails are trimmed short.

* Children with the condition should wear underpants or knickers under their night clothes to try and prevent hand contact with the anal region where they itch.

* Ensure that everyone routinely washes their hands thoroughly after using the toilet.

* Ensure that everyone, routinely washes their hands thoroughly before preparing food.

How should you treat threadworms?

Yourself:

If you see fine white threads on your child's stools after they have moved their bowels, or if you see fine threadworms at the entrance

127

THREADWORMS
'FILE O' FACTS'

* The cleanest household in the land can get threadworms.

* 1 in 4 children under 10 years has been infected at some stage.

* Threadworms do not come from animals or pets. They can only live in humans.

* The worms themselves are not contagious.

* The tiny eggs of the worm are easily passed on, as they are carried under fingernails, on skin and therefore on food, on clothes and on bedding.

* The female worm lays 10,000 eggs just outside the back passage, whilst the child is asleep. This causes intense itching.

* The child scratches his bottom, the eggs get onto the fingers and under the fingernails and are therefore, transferred easily to other people, and also back into the child's own mouth to re-infest the child again.

* Eggs can live outside the body on bedding, nightclothes, underwear, floors and walls for several weeks.

* A child with threadworms has caught them from someone else.

* 45% of the UK population has suffered from threadworm.

to your child's back passage (anus), you would be best advised to discuss this with your doctor. He will prescribe a treatment to kill the worms. This is known as an anthelminthic (see below).

GP:

Treatments available include the following:

* *Vermox*
* *Combantrin*
* *Pripsen*
* *Antepar*

Vermox is the treatment of choice. It is only available on prescription. The dosage for all children over 2 years and all adults is one teaspoonful (5ml) straight away and followed by another teaspoon 14–21 days afterwards.

All members of the family should:

* Receive the same treatment at both times, even though they do not show any signs of threadworm infestation.

* Keep finger nails short.

* Wash and scrub hands and finger nails with a nailbrush, after using the toilet and before preparing food.

* Disinfect the toilet handle, door handle and toilet seat often.

Alongside these recommendations, the affected child should:

* Have a bath every MORNING, washing the bottom in particular.

* Keep to his own towel.

* Regularly change underclothes, clothes and bedding.

The above recommendations MUST be adhered to for SIX WEEKS following the first dose of medicine.

A common reason for children becoming re-infected with threadworms again and again is that the above recommendations are not strictly adhered to.

ACCIDENTS
& EMERGENCIES

BROKEN BONES

Another name for a broken bone is a fracture.

Children, particularly those under 5 years, are prone to falls and all sorts of other incidents that can put them at risk of getting a broken bone. Sometimes it can be difficult to know whether your child has just sprained or twisted himself or whether he has actually suffered a break in a bone. This can be very worrying.

IF YOU ARE AT ALL WORRIED AFTER YOUR CHILD HAS HAD A FALL OR INJURY, CONTACT YOUR GP OR TAKE THE CHILD TO THE CASUALTY DEPARTMENT OF YOUR LOCAL HOSPITAL.

Is the bone broken?
The three classical signs of a fracture or broken bone are:
* Pain.
* Bruising.
* Abnormal shape or alignment.

Other helpful clues are:
* A crack was heard or felt.
* Inability to move affected part.
* Swelling and tenderness over the affected part.

Unfortunately, children don't always present with these classic symptoms. Because of their regular falls when learning to walk and their lack of knowledge of dangerous situations, Mother Nature has protected them with 'bendy' bones. A child's bones do not snap as easily as the hard bones of an adult. The bone often bends and only partially breaks like a twig might on bending. This is known as a 'greenstick' fracture. This name, in fact, tells you how the bone would break – just like the green sticks used by gardeners to prop up plants. The break does not go right across the shaft of the bone, and the bone tries to return back to its original shape, thus causing minimal damage to surrounding

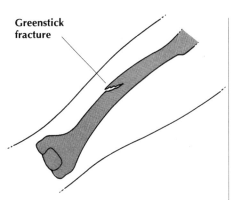

Greenstick fracture

nerves, blood vessels and muscles.

Your child might not show any deformity of the affected limb so the clues to look out for are pain, tenderness, an inability to move the limb and bruising.

What do you do?
If the bone is obviously bent:
* Dial 999 for an ambulance.
* DO NOT attempt to straighten it.
* KEEP YOUR HANDS OFF!
* Do not move the child.
* Don't give the child anything to eat or drink, as they may need a general anaesthetic.
* Stay with the child, calmly comforting him until help arrives.

If the bone is not bent:
* Try to support the affected part, e.g. for an arm use a

sling, for fingers tape them together, for legs don't even attempt to strap them together, call the ambulance.
* Take the child to Casualty, immediately, or call the ambulance.
* Do not give the child anything to eat or drink.

At hospital
Following an examination by the casualty doctor, the child will be X-rayed to give a clear picture of the bone and the extent of the injury. If the broken ends of the bone are close to each other and in a straight line the child's limb will probably be set in a plaster of Paris cast. If the bone ends are out of line the child will be given a general anaesthetic and the bones re-aligned in the right position for optimum healing. For more serious breaks your child may have to remain in hospital.

The plaster cast is removed once the bone has repaired itself. The child can then return to full normal activity - children are so resilient that they are often back to nearly full activity within a week of the fracture, even though they've got an arm in plaster!

Once your child is home try to

131

keep the plaster cast dry, if you can! You won't be able to keep it clean, especially when your child discovers the age-old custom of putting pen to plaster – plaster graffiti!

Most bones heal in 6–8 weeks, but you will be given full instructions as to when to return to the hospital clinic.

BURNS AND SCALDS

What are burns and scalds?
Burns are injuries produced by dry heat. Scalds are injuries produced by hot liquids.

Treatment is the same for both.

Can you prevent burns?
All children are inquisitive, and we cannot stop them exploring, but we can take precautions to reduce the chances of them accidentally burning themselves. We all know where the accidents can occur, and with a little thought many of the following dangerous situations can be prevented. There are ways you can prevent these accidental burns:

* A child pulling over a pan of hot soup, hot water or hot fat onto itself by reaching up to the cooker.

BURNS 'FILE O'FACTS'

* Each year about 20,000 children end up in casualty departments around the land with burns.

* Every year 100 children die as a result of severe burns.

* Deaths from burns are decreasing, due to less open fires, improved fire guards and flame resistant nightdresses.

* 70% of burns occur in children under 5 years of age.

* Poor housing, family stress and overcrowding put children more at risk of getting burns.

* Hands and fingers are most frequently burned, followed by face.

* House fires are most frequently the result of smokers' items – cigarettes or matches.

* Touching an iron that has been left to cool.
* Touching the elements of an electric fire.
* Touching hot surfaces such as open ovens, ceramic hobs, convection heaters, fan heaters.
* Knocking a cup of hot tea or coffee over a child.
* Playing with matches and cigarettes (copying adults).
* Unsafe fire-guards or even unguarded open fires. Remember bouncing, colourful flames are fascinating to an inquisitive toddler.
* A toddler unable to see that the cord he is pulling off the kitchen work surface is attached to a kettle of boiling water.

How should you treat burns and scalds?
With all burns or scalds SPEED of treatment is the most important factor. The sooner you react and DO THE RIGHT THING the better chance your child has of avoiding serious damage and possible scarring.

* Put the burn under COLD water – AT ONCE. Keep the cold water running for at least 10 minutes. Your child may not like this as cold water can be uncomfortable, but not as uncomfortable as a painful disfiguring burn. In extensive burns plunge the child under a cool shower or into a cool bath. You have to COOL that hot skin RAPIDLY.
* DON'T use butter or oils on a burn, they don't cool it enough and they are difficult to clean from the burn afterwards.
* DON'T prick any blisters, you may introduce infection.
* Cover the burn with a clean handkerchief or pillow-case, soaked in cold water, or cling-film and get the child to hospital IMMEDIATELY.
* Only the smallest of burns should be treated at home.
* Paracetamol will relieve the pain, as will raising the affected part.

Electric burns
If your child has suffered an electric shock:

* Immediately switch off the appliance. If this cannot be done do NOT attempt to pull him off because if the

133

appliance is still connected to the electricity supply you will receive an electric shock. In that situation try to separate him from the live wire or appliance by pushing him away with a non-conducting object such as a wooden broom, chair or stool. If you are standing on newspapers that will insulate you from the ground and reduce your chances of getting a shock.

* After separating him from the live current, treat any burns as outlined above.
* Lay your child down, elevate his legs and turn his head to one side. This will prevent shock and also prevent him inhaling vomit if he is sick
* If he is unconscious, lie him face down with his .

head turned to one side. The ideal 'recovery' position is demonstrated here (see diagram below).

* Call the ambulance on 999

Fire and flames
If your child's clothing has caught fire:

* Stop him running around in a panic – this will fan the flames and make matters worse.
* Throw him or force him to the ground, so that he is flat. This stops the flames rising to his upper body and face.
* Throw water over the flames (but not if your child is still connected to an electrical appliance) or smother the flames in towels, coats, curtains or whatever you can get your hands on.
* Treat any burns as directed above.
* Call the ambulance on 999

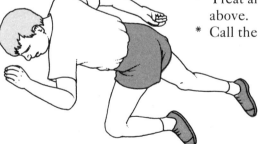

Recovery position

134

CHOKING

Although choking is a rare occurrence, every parent should know how to deal with this emergency in three categories of children:

* babies
* small children
* older children

The principles are simple and similar for all age groups. If you don't get it right first time, you won't get a second chance. It's a dire emergency that can kill – YOU could save your child's life!

Children are more at risk of choking because they're always putting things into their mouths and even with food they may not chew it adequately. Fortunately these situations don't happen very often, but if they do they are absolute EMERGENCIES, as anything inhaled into the windpipe can totally block the airways and halt breathing. Parents concerned about these rare, but potentially lethal occurrences could obtain full practical training in resuscitation and first aid techniques from the St John's Ambulance people. They will be listed in your local telephone directory.

What are the signs of choking?

* The child may have a coughing fit.
* He grasps at his throat.
* He fights for his breath, making croaking noises.
* His face turns blue.

What do you do to stop choking?

ACT IMMEDIATELY

Babies

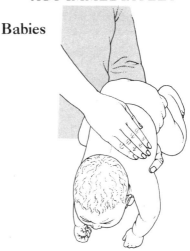

1. Quickly lay baby face down on your forearm, with his head lower than his bottom.

2. Give him several hard slaps between the shoulder blades.

3. As soon as the object is dislodged get it out of his mouth immediately, taking care not to push it back down the throat.

Small children

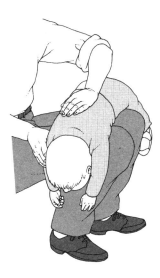

Older children

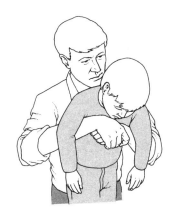

1. With the child standing, get behind him and put your arms around his lower chest.

1. Quickly lay the child face down over your lap, with his head lower than his bottom.

2. Give him several hard slaps between the shoulder blades on the upper part of his back.

3. As soon as the object is dislodged, get it out of his mouth immediately, taking care not to push it back down the throat.

2. Put one fist under his ribs in the midline. Place the other hand over the fist and thrust in and upwards very firmly.

3. Repeat until the object is dislodged, then get him to spit it out.

This technique is called the Heimlich manoeuvre and can also be used with adults.

WHILST PERFORMING ANY OF THESE ACTIONS GET SOMEONE ELSE TO DIAL 999 IMMEDIATELY FOR AN AMBULANCE. This is to ensure that expert help is quickly available in case you are not successful in dislodging the object.

Even if you are successful at dislodging the object, you should still seek medical advice straight away.

CUTS AND GRAZES

Cuts

Any cut that is bleeding should have pressure directly applied to the cut itself with a clean gauze or handkerchief. In an emergency any cloth will do, dirty or clean! Direct pressure, if possible, is the best way to stop bleeding in any part of the body. Pressure may have to be applied for about 5 minutes, which seems an eternity at the time!

Once bleeding has stopped, clean the area with antiseptic – it will sting if it gets into the cut. Very small cuts can be covered with adhesive dressings, making sure that the edges of the cut are closely aligned to each other. If there is any uncertainty about tetanus protection in your child, call your doctor for advice.

If you are unsure whether the cut should be stitched, or if bleeding cannot be controlled, contact your GP or take the child to Casualty. Any cuts on the face or cuts that may be deep should be looked at by a doctor, especially if there is a possibility of a foreign body, such as glass, being in the wound.

Stitches, or sutures as the doctor calls them, will usually be removed by your GP or the hospital, 5–7 days after they've been put in.

HINT

A couple of days before your child is to have his stitches taken out, gently soak them in soapy water twice a day, morning and evening. This helps to soften the blood clots and crusts that have formed over the cut and around the stitches. These crusts or scabs then come away and make the removal of the stitches far less uncomfortable for the child and a much quicker process. It can be very painful for a child to have a doctor trying to dig the stitches out of a thick layer of coagulated old blood.

Grazes

These should be cleaned with water, or antiseptic liquid if your child will tolerate the stinging effect! Try to remove any particles of grit and, if possible, leave open to the air - this helps a dry crust to form on the surface of the graze, which then speeds up the healing beneath.

If the graze becomes infected apply an antiseptic cream, or your doctor might prescribe an antibiotic cream, along with a dressing such as *Melolin* which will help the healing. Remember to apply the plastic side of the dressing next to the skin – the gauze side would stick to the graze causing great distress to the frightened little patient when removing the dressing.

HEAD INJURY

Children are always falling and banging themselves – it's a wonder so many reach adulthood free of serious injury!

Thankfully most bangs to the head make the child cry, feel very upset for a short while and then the child is back playing with his friends.

However, there are circumstances when a bang to the head can be more serious and then you need to know what to do.

BANGS TO THE HEAD

Any of the following symptoms occurring in a child who has had a bang to the head, need urgent medical attention. In these circumstances, take your child to the nearest casualty department or call your GP or an ambulance immediately.

* An unconscious child.
* Vomiting
* Persistent headache.
* Drowsiness.
* Blurred or double vision.
* Bleeding from nose or ear.
* Pale yellow fluid from nose or ear.

Even if some of these symptoms happen 12–24 hours after a head injury you must still get medical attention for the child.

If your child has an open wound that is bleeding, apply direct pressure to the wound itself with a handkerchief or clean pad until medical help arrives.

An unconscious child MUST be put into the 'recovery position', until help arrives (see page 134).

POISONING

* In the under 5 year-olds, accidental poisoning is one of the commonest reasons for children seeking emergency medical treatment at hospital.

* Coloured tablets, medicines, alcohol, detergents, disinfectants, chemicals, plants and berries are some of the poisonous substances children will commonly ingest, as a result of their enquiring minds!

* If you suspect that your child has swallowed any possibly poisonous substance contact your doctor IMMEDIATELY. If he is not available
either
  – ring the casualty department of your local hospital, they will be able to give you precise advice on what to do,
or
  – call an ambulance on 999.

Take any containers that may be relevant to the accidental poisoning with you to the doctor or hospital.

* NEVER try to induce vomiting in a child that is known to have taken bleach, disinfectant, paraffin, petrol or any other chemical. Vomiting may rupture a stomach or gullet already corroded by the chemical!

* Suspect accidental poisoning in any child who:
  – starts vomiting for no obvious reason.
  – becomes drowsy, confused or loses consciousness.
  – starts breathing erratically.

* Look for clues of berries, tablets, etc. close to the child.

STINGS

The most common stings in this country are from bees and wasps. They are usually not serious, just painful, swollen, red and itchy.

What do you do?
Keep calm. If you panic your child will be even more frightened.

See if the sting is still in the skin. If it is, don't pull it out with your

139

fingers. In doing this you will probably squeeze the little bag of poison that is still attached to the sting, and inject more of the poison into your child!

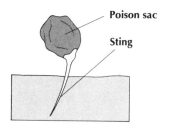

Poison sac

Sting

Remove the sting by scraping it off the skin surface with your fingernail or a knife blade.

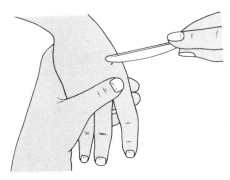

Compress the part with a cloth soaked in cold water, and then gently apply a good layer of hydrocortisone cream. Try to keep the affected part elevated to ease the pain and if necessary give the child some paracetamol.

Hydrocortisone cream should be in every first aid kit as it is now available from the chemist without a doctor's prescription. It is very useful for insect bites and stings, nettle stings, allergic skin reactions and sunburn.

Anaphylactic (*anna-fill-aktik*) shock

In very rare situations some people are extremely sensitive to wasp or bee stings. They have developed an allergic reaction through having been stung once before, and this exaggerated or hypersensitive reaction can be life threatening. The symptoms include:

* Difficulty in breathing, due to closing of the throat.
* Rapid onset of swelling of the eyes, face and mouth.
* Intense itching all over the body.

These may then be followed by the symptoms of shock:

* Going pale.
* Sweating.
* Cold, clammy skin.
* Fast, feeble pulse.
* Feeling faint.

If ever this type of reaction is encountered ring 999 for an ambulance – THIS IS AN EMERGENCY SITUATION!

INDEX

141

*The Smoker's Quit
Plan* by Dr Chris
Steele (£3.50) is
available from:
Gardiner-Caldwell
Communications
The Old Ribbon
Mill, Pitt St,
Macclesfield,
Cheshire
SK11 7PT